LUPUS DIET COOKBOOK

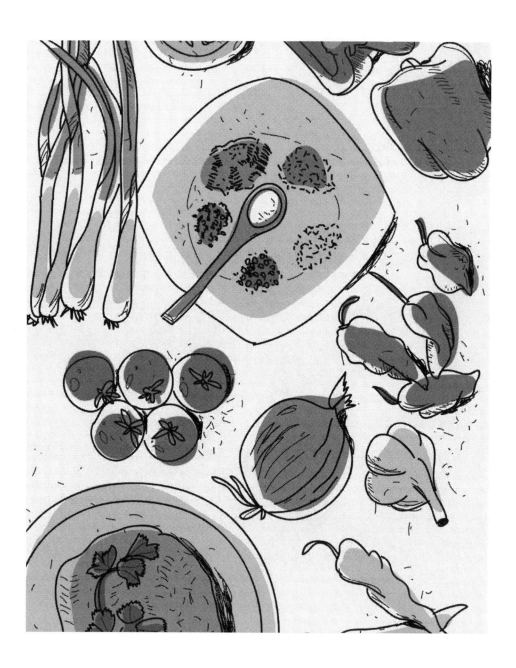

Lupus

Diet

Cookbook

Top 100 Lupus Diet Recipes to Reduce Inflammation and Live Your Best Life with Lupus

Karen Willard

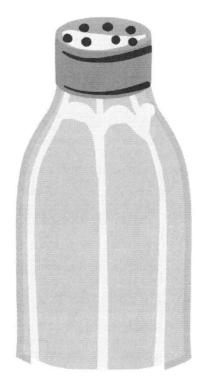 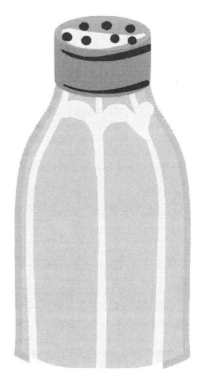

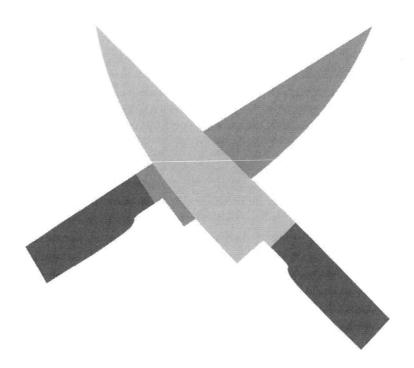

6

CONTENTS

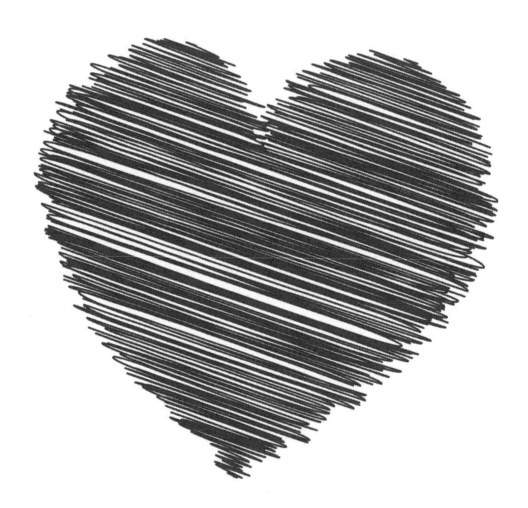

MY LIFE WITH LUPUS AND HOW AN ANTI-INFLAMMATORY DIET HELPED ME

My name is Karen and I was diagnosed with systemic lupus erythematosus six years ago. I have been a healthy individual ever since, which is why everyone, including myself, were surprised when laboratory tests confirmed that I have the condition. I later realized that I was actually living a stress-filled life, especially when I started working, got married, and became a mom.

Before cooking became my life I was a salesperson, and if you're familiar with sales, you know just how high the level of stress is involved in that line of work. For years, I spent my life dealing with high levels of stress. Even when I tried to leave work at the office, I couldn't, and that made matters worse, since I also had to deal with things at home with my husband and two kids.

The first couple years following my diagnoses were very miserable. If not for the support of my family and friends and my doctor, I don't know what would have happened to me. Of course, I also received comfort from other lupus patients whom I've met along the way, some of whom have eventually become very good friends of mine.

It was from one of these friends that I've learned about the AI diet or the anti-inflammatory diet. She told me that I should try it as it really helped her manage her symptoms. I told myself, "Why not? If it worked for her, perhaps it would work for me, too."

I didn't just jump into right away, though. I committed to two weeks of researching and learning all I can about this so-called anti-inflammatory diet. I read books about it, thoroughly surfed the net for articles and studies that supported its claims, and of course, asked for advice from my doctor and dietician. They both gave me the go signal and the rest was history.

I started avoiding foods that were rich in starch and carbohydrates. According to books and articles I've read, high-starch foods are difficult to digest and that people with compromised immune systems may not respond very well to such foods. I also stopped buying and eating processed foods and eliminated from my diet anything that contained gluten, gran, lactose, processed sugar, and anything that contained components that are harder for the digestive system to break down, and often cause inflammation.

And then I focused on eating whole foods, lots of fruits and vegetables, and fish. I ate chicken and lean beef from time to time, although much of my diet was just mainly leafy greens and plant-based proteins. After only a few months of following this eating plan, I noticed significant changes in my body. I began to regain my normal weight. I also noticed that I had more energy than usual. I still visited my doctor regularly and made sure I continued living a healthy lifestyle, exercising as much as I can and avoiding anything that may worsen my symptoms.

I was glad that my doctor, as well as my family and friends kept on supporting me. It's been several years now since I started following an anti-inflammatory eating plan, and I would say that it has really helped me manage my lupus symptoms. Yes, I still have lupus, but I would say that I have never felt better in my life.

I'm not saying that following an AI diet is going to cure your lupus or any health condition you may have, but I can assure you that it's going to change your life. It may not cure everything that is ailing you right now, but it's going to help you heal, and that's the most important thing.

Yours in Good Health,

Karen Willard

WHAT IS LUPUS?

Lupus is an autoimmune disease, which means it causes the body's immune system to become hyperactive and attack normal, healthy cells. Normally, it's the immune system that protects the body against infection and illness. In the case of lupus, however, the immune system attacks instead of protects bodily tissues. This anomalous activity of the immune system causes damage to tissues and results in illness. Lupus is a long-term disease and is characterized by swelling and inflammation, as well as damage to the skin, joints, blood, and organs like the heart, kidney, and lungs.

According to statistics from the Lupus Foundation of America, about 1.5 million U.S. residents have lupus. However, individuals of Native American, Asian, and African descent are those who are more likely to develop the condition. And although lupus does not respect gender, 90% of those diagnosed with the said disease are females, particularly those who are between 14 to 45 years of age.

WHAT CAUSES LUPUS?

It's unclear how a person acquires lupus, but the cause may either be genetic, hormonal, environmental, or a combination of the three.

Lupus is more common in some families, although researchers haven't proven yet that lupus may be caused by some genetic factor. One reason genetics is considered when talking of lupus causes, however, is that the disease is up to three times more common in people of color than in caucasians. In the same manner, an individual who has a relative with lupus have a higher chance of developing the condition, too.

Scientists have already identified certain genes that may play a part in the development of the disease, but there's no adequate proof that they can indeed cause lupus. What's clear, though, is that individuals with no family history of lupus can acquire it. Although, it may be because there are other types of autoimmune diseases, such as hemolytic anemia and thyroiditis in the family.

Meanwhile, the U.S. National Institutes of Health says that females are more likely to have lupus than males, with a risk that's nine times higher. On this percentage, it is suspected by researchers that there may be a link between the hormone estrogen and lupus. In a 2016 study, it has been discovered that estrogen can induce lupus antibodies, although this was observed not in humans but in mice that are susceptible to the disease. This may explain why females are more likely to acquire lupus and other autoimmune diseases than men.

Environmental agents, too, have been found to be a possible contributor to lupus. Chemicals and viruses are said to have the potential to trigger lupus in individuals who are genetically susceptible to the disease. Smoking, in particular, is considered a possible culprit in the rise in the number of lupus cases in that past few decades. Medication is also a culprit, possibly contributing to ten percent of cases.

What is perhaps the most interesting recent find by scientists is the possibility of microbe population living in the gut (the intestines, in particular) being a factor in the development of lupus. In 2018, a research published in Applied and Environmental Microbiology found distinct changes in the gut microbe population in individuals with lupus. The same has been discovered in mice that have the condition. While the researchers recommended more research to be done in this area, it is clear that what happens in the gut has a direct link to lupus.

NO CURE FOR LUPUS

Lupus, like most types of autoimmune diseases, has no cure. One moment it flares up, and another moment it disappears, only to appear again with no warning. The only thing that can be done with lupus is to manage its symptoms. It is usually achieved with a combination of certain medications and changes in diet and lifestyle. In addition, regular visits to the doctor and lab tests are necessary to find out whether or not the treatment is taking effect and if there are any potential side effects. For mild lupus, treatment usually requires monitoring every 6 months to a year.

DIET IS THE KEY

When it comes to managing symptoms of lupus, diet is always one of the keys. Again, one of the main symptoms of lupus is swelling, which is a result of inflammation. Inflammation in itself is not bad since it's a natural process that helps the body protect itself from harm and even heal and recover from infection. The problem, however, is when inflammation becomes chronic.

Chronic inflammation is the prolonged inflammatory response of the body that involves a progressive change in the cells found at the inflammation site. Overtime, it may lead to a number of health problems. It is characterized by a simultaneous breaking down and repair of the tissue. While symptoms of lupus may vary from person to person, inflammation is usually present, whether in the form of arthritis, arthralgia, swelling of the ankles, and the like. For people with lupus, a key factor in managing symptoms is the prevention of inflammation with the help of an anti-inflammatory diet.

There's no questioning the negative effects of inflammation as there's a good number of research that has proven it. Alzheimer's, cancer, obesity[1] -- all of these and similar chronic diseases[2] are linked to inflammation. Several other studies have also looked at the implications of following a diet that's rich in anti-inflammatory foods on certain medical conditions. One study, for instance, has shown that eating more anti-inflammatory foods may help those suffering from rheumatoid arthritis.[3] Now, while an AI diet may not necessarily cure you if you have any health condition, it may help reduce the impact of certain diseases by delaying their progression. It may even help reduce the amount of medication you will need in some cases.

You need to understand that despite what others might say, there's no specific diet that people with lupus should follow. An important thing to keep in mind when dealing with lupus is for one to eat a healthy, balanced diet of fresh fruits and vegetables, plant fat, legumes, whole grains, fish, and lean protein.

---

[1] https://www.ncbi.nlm.nih.gov/pmc/articles/PMC3583126/
[2] https://www.ncbi.nlm.nih.gov/pmc/articles/PMC3170500/
[3] https://www.ncbi.nlm.nih.gov/pmc/articles/PMC5682732/

However, while that is the case, there are certain foods that are better than others for helping you manage lupus symptoms. This is where a diet of anti-inflammatory foods come in.

THE IMPORTANCE OF AN ANTI-INFLAMMATORY DIET FOR LUPUS

Again, inflammation within the body is not a bad thing. In fact, it's the immune's system's way of protecting the body. When you're having an inflammation, it means your immune system is sending out white blood cells and compounds to fight off whatever's threatening you, whether it's toxins, bacteria, or viruses. Normal inflammation is characterized by pain, redness, heat, and swelling around the area that has been injured or wounded. Think of a minor sprain on your ankle, for instance.

Now, there's another response called 'resolution' designed to heal damaged tissues. The first stage of inflammation results in the destruction of the cells. The second stage, which is resolution, is when cellular rejuvenation takes place. The body remains well as long as the balance between these stages is retained.

Unfortunately, this is not always the case for many people. The balance isn't achieved and that as a result of what enters an individual's stomach. Refined grains, sugar, and saturated fat, all trigger an inflammatory response from the immune system. The fact that our diet nowadays are usually filled with the abovementioned elements doesn't help because every time you eat fast food or any kind of food containing high amounts of sugar, bad fats, and the like, you are causing inflammation on different parts of your body over and over.

Not only that, but people nowadays don't get enough fruits and vegetables that are jam-packed with antioxidants and possess anti-inflammatory properties. Most of us don't get to eat enough fatty fish, too, which is actually an excellent source of omega-3 fatty acids. If you don't know it yet, omega-3 facilitates in the moving of the body into the rejuvenating or resolution stage.

Of course, there are other factors that trigger the immune system to respond in this manner. Take air pollution, for instance. Environmental toxins, too. Among these factors, however, it is our diet that has the most impact on inflammation. Eating food high in bad cholesterol, for instance, can cause inflammation of the arteries, which leads to heart problems.

In the joints, this same inflammation results in pain and swelling. In the digestive system, inflammation causes the elimination of good bacteria and damages the lining of the intestines. This contributes to irritable bowel syndrome, and even obesity. In the brain, inflammation manifests in the form of anxiety and even depression. Lupus, which is characterized by swelling and inflammation, is also said to be a result of poor eating habits.

On the contrary, research shows that following an anti-inflammatory diet has the potential to reduce the risk of heart diseases, obesity, and even some forms of cancer. Scientists even claim that it may extend life. There is not much evidence yet, but some experts also claim that anti-inflammatory diet, particularly the extreme ones, may help reverse autoimmune disease (like lupus!), as well as improve mental health. Again, however, there is still a lot more research that needs to be done to prove this claim.

What Does An Anti-Inflammatory Diet Look Like?

Unlike most popular diets, such as the South Beach diet, for instance, there is no specific anti-inflammatory diet. In fact, there are several diets that have been around for some time now that can be considered an anti-inflammatory diet or AI. The Mediterranean diet and the DASH diet both would score well in terms of being anti-inflammatory. Even the Paleo and the Whole30 diets can be classified as AI.

Among these diets, however, the one that's most backed by research when it comes to being AI is the Mediterranean diet. You've probably heard of this plan inspired by the eating habits of those living in Italy and Greece. It emphasizes the consumption of fruits and vegetables, whole grains and legumes, and fish and olive oil. A number of studies confirm this, claiming that people who observe the Mediterranean style of eating have lower C-reactive protein and interleukin-6 levels, both of which are inflammatory markers.[4]

According to one study, the lower levels of C-reactive protein or CRP are linked to a high consumption of fruits, vegetables, fish, and some dairy products. This is one of the reasons the Mediterranean diet is placed on top of all other diets as the best diet overall. For many people, adhering to this type of diet has resulted in loss of excess weight, as well as lowering of risks for heart problems and stroke.

The AI diet has one simple goal, and that is to eliminate foods that trigger inflammatory response and consume more foods that facilitate tissue repair. Since there isn't one specific AI eating plan, there aren't any strict rules when it comes to what's allowed and what isn't. However, a true AI plan always highlights the importance of eating whole, unprocessed foods, monounsaturated fats (those found in olive oil, berries, avocados, and other fruits), and omega-3 fatty acids from fish like tuna, salmon, mackerel. It also emphasizes on avoided refined grains and food rich in added sugar.

With that, it's important to note that even if your friend or colleague at work is following an AI like you, it doesn't necessarily mean that your plate will look the same. But that's how AI diet works. Different people have different needs. A grain-free diet may work for you and not for another person. Your friend may not hesitate to give up bread but you believe you can't live without it and that's perfectly okay.

Aside from the fact that you're unique, food sensitivities also have a role to play here. People react to food differently. If you have a sensitivity to a particular type of food, eating that food may lead to production of cytokine, as well as an increase in the amount of various inflammatory chemicals in your body.

It may sound cheesy and cliche, but you must think of an AI diet as a lifestyle and not just a diet. The AI diet works by reducing low-grade inflammation with the body, but you can't achieve results unless you take it seriously. Nutritionists agree that the ideal serving of fruits and veggies is at least seven per day. AI also requires that you limit your intake of meat (red meat, in particular) and dairy, and replace simple carbohydrates with complex carbohydrates. Finally, it demands that you eliminate processed foods from your diet. That's not something that can easily be done without self-discipline, but if you have lupus or any similar medical condition, it makes a lot of sense to stick to an AI diet regardless of what it takes.

---

[4] https://www.ncbi.nlm.nih.gov/pmc/articles/PMC5872797/

COMPELLING REASONS TO FOLLOW AN ANTI-INFLAMMATORY DIET IF YOU HAVE LUPUS

Whether or not you're suffering from chronic inflammation as a result of medical conditions like lupus, it makes sense to follow an anti-inflammatory diet. It is a way of life and will surely improve your health in the end. Anyone can benefit from such a diet plan as AI, and there is so much proof that it is helpful for people with chronic inflammation or are suffering from any health condition. The following are just some of the many reasons you should try this eating plan:

It Will Make You Feel Full Much Longer

The anti-inflammatory diet is packed with pulses, superfoods you've probably never heard of. Pulses are actually those dried edible seeds found on certain plants belonging to the legume family. They are rich in antioxidants and minerals that are not only essential to everyday life, but are necessary if you are to fight off inflammation. This food group includes lentils, chickpeas, beans, and dry peas, and are a rich source of protein, fiber, vitamins, and minerals. Despite their size, they can count toward your recommended daily chunk of fruits and vegetables. Combining fiber, unsaturated fats, and lean protein, pulses can fill you up without affecting your diet.

It Will Boost Your Mood

Having a clear mind is crucial when you're dealing with a condition like lupus. Living with lupus can be challenging. Symptoms come and go, and you never really know what each day will bring. With such a condition, it's normal to experience anger, frustration, and feelings of sadness. This is one area an anti-inflammatory diet can help. A major component of an anti-inflammatory diet is fish, particularly those that are high in omega-3 content. 12 ounces a week of fish rich in omega-3s is enough to provide you with a ton of anti-inflammatory benefits. Anchovies, salmon, sardines, tuna, plus other types of white fish are all packed with omega-3 fatty acids, which have been linked to reduced anxiety symptoms and a lower risk of depression.[5]

It May Help You Lose Some Weight

It's not uncommon for individuals with lupus to acquire autoimmune thyroid problems. When the thyroid isn't functioning well, organs like the brain, heart, liver, and kidneys are often affected. It also results in weight problems. Following an AI diet doesn't necessarily mean you will lose weight, especially if you have a healthy weight to begin with. Nevertheless, there's always a huge chance that a diet rich in vegetables and low in refined carbs and sugar will help you meet your weight loss goals. As mentioned, an AI diet will make you feel fuller even just on a few calories because of the volume of the fiber-rich foods that compose it.

It's An Inclusive And Not An Exclusive Eating Plan

If you've had lupus for some time now, you're probably already tired of hearing what you can't put on your plate during meal times. With an anti-inflammatory diet, more is better. This doesn't mean you can eat whatever you want. One advantage of an AI diet over traditional diets is that it's more inclusive than

---

[5] https://www.health.harvard.edu/blog/omega-3-fatty-acids-for-mood-disorders-2018080314414

exclusive. With that, it means the focus is not on what you can't and shouldn't eat but on what you're supposed to eat. For an AI diet, colorful foods are a top priority. Leafy greens like kale and spinach, cruciferous like cauliflower and broccoli, carotenoids like carrots and tomatoes, and anthocyanins that include berries and beets are all a staple in an anti-inflammatory diet.

WHAT FOOD IS IN AN ANTI-INFLAMMATORY DIET?

The exact description of the anti-inflammatory diet varies depending on who's describing, although it's probably closest to the Mediterranean Diet. It's also similar to the Zone diet, except that it doesn't exclude fish oil. If you want to follow an anti-inflammatory diet for your lupus, you need to be prepared to load up on foods that according to studies have been found to lower inflammation. You also need to be prepared to cut back on foods that promote the opposite effect.

The best thing about an AI diet is that the food options are actually very plenty. There's also a lot of wiggle room, which means you're not limited to foods you like less. On the contrary, it leaves you plenty of room to choose those types of food that you like best. If you're the type of person who needs more structure, then the Mediterranean diet should work for you since there's a lot of overlap between it and the anti-inflammatory diet. Both emphasizes eating lots of whole grains, as well as plenty of fruits and vegetables.

Speaking of which, fresh fruits, including grapes, grapefruit, bananas, blueberries, and apples are a staple of an AI diet. Mangoes, peaches, and pomegranates are included in the list, as well.

- Dried Fruits (dates, dlums, prunes, apricots, cranberries)
- Vegetables (broccoli, brussels sprouts, cauliflower)
- Leafy Greens (spinach, kale, romaine lettuce)
- Plant-Based Proteins (lentils, seitan, chickpeas, spirulina)
- Whole Grains (brown rice, oatmeal, sorghum, whole wheat bread, quinoa)
- Nuts (almonds, walnuts, pistachios, peanuts)
- Seeds (flaxseeds, chia seeds, sesame seeds, pumpkin seeds)
- Spices (black pepper, cayenne, cinnamon, clove, ginger, turmeric)
- Fatty Fish (salmon, tuna, mackerel, herring, sardines, lake trout)
- Coffee, green tea, dark chocolate, and red wine in moderation

These are simply food suggestions. You don't have to follow any anti-inflammatory diet perfectly to achieve the best results. A healthy immune system is designed to handle the periodic assault of inflammation, like when you're having that piece of cake at your friend's birthday party. What's not good is the regular and consistent consumption of sugary foods and foods rich in saturated fat. These are inflammatory foods, and when overconsumed, can lead to serious problems.

The key, therefore, is not to focus on a super diet, but on the individual foods. If you're regularly eating anti-inflammatory foods and yet often eat a bunch of inflammatory foods at the same time, you're still not doing yourself any favor. On most days, you should follow these guidelines to maximize your effort:

1. Aim for at least half of your meal to be non-starchy veggies. This includes most leafy greens, squash, beets, cauliflower, and even mushroom. They're jam packed with antioxidants and fiber that are essential for gut health.

2. Cut back on sugary foods and drinks. This includes honey, which is a natural sweetener, as well as most types of fruit juices. While these may seem beneficial for the health, they can also increase haptoglobin in the blood, an inflammatory marker that when in very high levels can lead to diabetes, obesity, heart attack, and stroke.

3. Eat a lot of fish. Again, fish like anchovies, herring, mackerel, and salmon, are rich in omega-3 fatty acids. If you can't consume such fish regularly, take at least 1,000 mg of omega-3 supplements daily.

4. Eliminate flour-based foods. Instead, focus on whole grains like brown rice and quinoa. Bread, crackers, and the like can cause a blood sugar spike that worsens inflammation. This is especially true if you have diabetes or are insulin resistant.

5. Limit saturated fats. The immune system sees meat rich in saturated fats as a threat because they contain the same fatty acids that are found on most bacteria. Butter, vegetable oil, corn oils, and oils abundant in omega-6 fats -- these are not good for you and can exacerbate inflammation. Aim for olive oil instead, as well as avocado and walnut oil.

FOODS TO EAT SPARINGLY IN AN AI DIET

I've mentioned that the best part about an AI diet is that it is not a totally restrictive kind of diet. When you're dealing with a condition like lupus, however, there is not one type of eating plan that works. That said, while most foods in an AI diet are okay for healthy people, there are some foods that are not for people with lupus or similar condition.

For a regular AI diet, foods to avoid or eat sparingly basically include the following:

- Refined carbs (white bread, sweets, pastries)
- Sugar-rich food and drinks (soda, fruit juice, spaghetti sauce, flavored coffee)
- Dairy (milk, cheese, yogurt, ice cream)
- Processed meat (hotdogs, sausages, corned beef, beef jerky, lunch meats, bacon)
- Red meat (beef, lamb, pork, goat, venison, veal)
- Fried foods (french fries, onion rings, hushpuppies)

Some of these are totally not good for lupus, while others, like yogurt, cheese, and low-fat milk are okay when consumed sparingly. Dairy, for instance, may help with lupus as a means of providing you with more calcium. This is especially true if you are taking medication that can thin the bones. Steroid medication, in particular, can affect bone health and may cause you to be more vulnerable to fractures and injuries. Eating foods rich in calcium will help offset this side effect.

With lupus, one of your top goals should be to follow a diet that is low in trans fats and saturated fats. Some medication can increase your appetite and make you gain weight fast. In that case, you will need to carefully watch what you eat. Avoid or limit trans and saturated fats and instead focus on foods that will help you feel full without actually filling you out, such as raw vegetables, fruits, and whole grains.

On Some Spices and Nightshade Vegetables

Other types of food that are included in an AI diet but are not okay if you have lupus are garlic and alfalfa. While garlic contain the anti-inflammatory compound diallyl disulfide, it also contains allicin, ajoene, and thiosulfinates, all of which can cause your lupus symptoms to flare up by sending your immune system into overdrive. Alfalfa, on the other hand, contain the amino acid L-canavanine, which, like allicin and company, can stimulate the immune system and increase inflammation.

The same is true with some nightshade vegetables. There isn't any scientific proof that such foods are bad for lupus, but some claim that they are sensitive to eggplant, tomatoes, white potatoes, cayenne pepper, bell pepper, and paprika. If you're not sure whether or not you have sensitivities to said foods, see to it that you keep a record of what you eat. Eliminate any type of food that you believe is causing your symptoms to flare up. This includes vegetables.

What About Salt?

Lupus already puts a person at higher risk for developing heart problems. If you have lupus, you may want to pass on salt, as eating an excess can cause your blood pressure to shoot up and increase your heart disease risk. It's true that your food won't be as flavorful without salt, but there are other spices you can use as substitute like lemon, herbs, curry powder, turmeric, and pepper.

It's also important to be vigilant when you're eating at a restaurant. To make sure your meal has less sodium in it, inform the server that you would want your meal to be served with little or no salt. And if possible, order an extra side of vegetables. Most veggies are rich in potassium, which can help combat the effects of sodium and lower blood pressure.

On Alcohol Intake

An occasional glass of wine or beer is fine when in moderate amounts. However, there are instances that alcohol might interact with medications you take for lupus. For instance, if you're taking ibuprofen and similar NSAID drugs, drinking alcohol may put you at risk of developing an ulcer. It can also hinder the effects of some medication and even increase their side effects. To be on the safe side, drink pure water or at least those that are mostly water like tea, diluted fruit juice, and sparkling water with lemon throughout the day.

ADDITIONAL THINGS TO CONSIDER

If it's not possible for you to eat fatty fish at least a couple times a week, you can substitute it with supplemental fish oil, whether in liquid or capsule form. Two to three times a day of supplements that contain EPA and DHA should be enough. Just make sure to opt for products that have been certified to be free of contaminants and heavy metals.

Speaking of oil, opt for extra-virgin oil as your main cooking oil as much as possible. Organic canola oil and organic sunflower or safflower oil are also okay if you're looking for something that's neutral-tasting.

Avoid margarine at all cost, as well as vegetable shortening, including any product that may list them as ingredients. Avoid products that contain partially hydrogenated oils, as well. Instead, add more to your diet avocados and nuts, especially almonds, walnuts, and cashews.

Finally, in choosing produce, go for organic whenever possible. Find out which conventionally grown crops are most likely to have been sprayed with pesticides and stay away from them. For your protein needs, eat more veggie proteins, especially from beans. Familiarize yourself with whole-soy foods and identify the ones you prefer.

In summary, following an anti-inflammatory diet is one of the keys to dealing with lupus. Lupus affects each individual differently, though, so a diet change that works for one may not work for another. Just remember that in following an anti-inflammatory diet, your main aim is variety. You also must include as much fresh foods to your meals as possible, and see to it that you stop or at least minimize your consumption of processed foods. More importantly, make it a habit of eating an abundance of fresh fruits and vegetables.

One way to get the most of an anti-inflammatory diet if you have lupus is to keep a food journal and to maintain transparent communication with your dietitian and your doctor. This will help you stay aware of which foods are good for you and which ones exacerbate your symptoms.

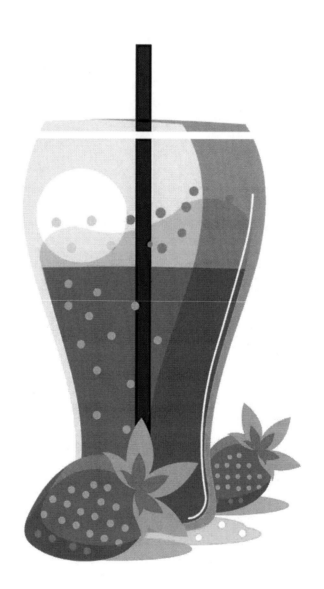

SMOOTHIE & BREAKFAST RECIPES

Contents

Banana & Spinach Smoothie

Serves: 2 / Preparation time: 10 minutes

1 frozen banana, peeled and sliced

1 tablespoon chia seeds

Pinch of ground cinnamon

½ cup ice cubes

2½ cups fresh baby spinach

1 tablespoon almond butter

1½ cups unsweetened almond milk

- In a high-speed blender, place all the ingredients and pulse until smooth.
- Place the smoothie into glasses and serve immediately

Per Serving: Calories: 155; Total Fat: 8.7g; Saturated Fat: 0.8g
Protein: 4.9g; Carbs: 19.5g; Fiber: 5.2g; Sugar: 7.7g

Peach Smoothie

Serves: 2 / Preparation time: 10 minutes

1½ cups frozen peaches, pitted and chopped   1 frozen banana, peeled and chopped

½ cup fat-free plain Greek yogurt   1 cup unsweetened almond milk

- In a high-speed blender, place all the ingredients and pulse until smooth.
- Place the smoothie into glasses and serve immediately

Per Serving: Calories: 144; Total Fat: 2.3g; Saturated Fat: 0.2g
Protein: 4.7g; Carbs: 29.2g; Fiber: 3.8g; Sugar: 17g

Mango Smoothie

Serves: 2 / Preparation time: 10 minutes

2 cups frozen mango, peeled, pitted and chopped

2 cups fresh spinach, chopped

1 tablespoon fresh lemon juice

16 ounces fresh coconut water

1 teaspoon ground turmeric

1 tablespoon fresh lime juice

- In a high-speed blender, place all the ingredients and pulse until smooth.
- Place the smoothie into glasses and serve immediately

Per Serving: Calories: 112; Total Fat: 0.9g; Saturated Fat: 0.3g
Protein: 2.4g; Carbs: 26.8g; Fiber: 3.6g; Sugar: 22g

Pineapple & Papaya Smoothie

Serves: 2 / Preparation time: 10 minutes

¾ cup pineapple, peeled and chopped

2 dates, pitted

¾ cup papaya, peeled and chopped

1½ cups fresh coconut water

- In a high-speed blender, place all the ingredients and pulse until smooth.
- Place the smoothie into glasses and serve immediately

Per Serving: Calories: 77; Total Fat: 0.3g; Saturated Fat: 0.1g
Protein: 0.8g; Carbs: 20.2g; Fiber: 2.5g; Sugar: 15.6g

Kale & Celery Smoothie

Serves: 2 / Preparation time: 10 minutes

1½ cups fresh kale, trimmed and chopped

½ of avocado, peeled, pitted and chopped

1 (½-inch) piece fresh turmeric root, peeled

2 cups chilled filtered water

2 celery stalks, chopped

1 (½-inch) piece fresh ginger root, peeled

1 teaspoon liquid stevia

- In a high-speed blender, place all the ingredients and pulse until smooth.
- Place the smoothie into glasses and serve immediately

Per Serving: Calories: 124; Total Fat: 9.9g; Saturated Fat: 2.1g
Protein: 2.1g; Carbs: 8.8g; Fiber: 4.2g; Sugar: 0.4g

Cucumber & Parsley Smoothie

Serves: 2 / Preparation time: 10 minutes

2 cups cucumber, peeled and chopped   1 cup fresh parsley

1 (1-inch) piece fresh ginger root, peeled and chopped

2 tablespoons fresh lemon juice   4-6 drops liquid stevia

2 cups chilled water

- In a high-speed blender, place all the ingredients and pulse until smooth.
- Place the smoothie into glasses and serve immediately

Per Serving: Calories: 31; Total Fat: 0.5g; Saturated Fat: 0.2g
Protein: 1.7g; Carbs: 6.1g; Fiber: 1.6g; Sugar: 2.3g

Herbed Greens Smoothie

Serves: 2 / Preparation time: 10 minutes

3 cups mixed fresh greens (spinach, kale, beet greens), trimmed and chopped

½ cup lettuce, torn

¼ cup fresh parsley leaves

¼ cup fresh mint leaves

2 tablespoons organic honey

1 tablespoon fresh lemon juice

1½ cups filtered water

¼ cup ice cubes

- In a high-speed blender, place all the ingredients and pulse until smooth.
- Place the smoothie into glasses and serve immediately

Per Serving: Calories: 102; Total Fat: 0.5g; Saturated Fat: 0.2g
Protein: 2g; Carbs: 25.2g; Fiber: 3.8g; Sugar: 18g

Green Veggies Smoothie

Serves: 2 / Preparation time: 10 minutes

2 cups fresh spinach

¼ cup green cabbage, chopped

2 cups chilled filtered water

¼ cup broccoli florets, chopped

6-8 drops liquid stevia

- In a high-speed blender, place all the ingredients and pulse until smooth.
- Place the smoothie into glasses and serve immediately

Per Serving: Calories: 13; Total Fat: 0.2g; Saturated Fat: 0g
Protein: 1.3g; Carbs: 2.4g; Fiber: 1.2g; Sugar: 0.6g

Mixed Fruit Yogurt Bowl

Serves: 2 / Preparation time: 15 minutes

1½ cups fat-free plain Greek yogurt

¼ cup peaches, pitted and chopped

¼ cup fresh blueberries

2 tablespoons almonds, chopped

2 tablespoons organic honey

¼ cup fresh raspberries

¼ cup fresh cherries, pitted

- In a large bowl, add yogurt and stevia and mix well.
- Add remaining ingredients and gently, stir to combine.
- Serve immediately.

Per Serving: Calories: 218; Total Fat: 3.4g; Saturated Fat: 0.2g
Protein: 9.6g; Carbs: 40.2g; Fiber: 2.9g; Sugar: 24g

Apple Porridge

Serves: 4 / Preparation time: 15 minutes / Cooking time: 4 minutes

2 cups unsweetened almond milk

3 tablespoons sunflower seeds

½ teaspoon organic vanilla extract

½ cup banana, peeled and sliced

2 large apples, peeled, cored and grated

¼ teaspoon ground cinnamon

½ cup fresh blueberries

¼ cup almonds, toasted and chopped

- In a large pan, add the almond milk, apples, sunflower seeds, cinnamon and vanilla extract and stir to combine.
- Place the pan over medium-low heat and cook for about 3-4 minutes, stirring occasionally.
- Remove from the heat and transfer into serving bowls.
- Set aside to cool slightly.
- Top with blueberries, banana slices and almonds and serve.

Per Serving: Calories: 154; Total Fat: 6.2g; Saturated Fat: 0.5g
Protein: 2.9g; Carbs: 25.2g; Fiber: 5.1g; Sugar: 16g

Spiced Chia Seeds Bowl

Serves: 4 / Preparation time: 15 minutes

1¾ cups unsweetened almond milk

1 tablespoon organic vanilla extract

2 (10-ounce) packages frozen raspberries, thawed

½ cup chia seeds

6 Medjool dates, pitted and chopped

- In a food processor, add all the ingredients except chia seeds and pulse until smooth.
- Transfer the mixture in a large bowl.
- Add the chia seeds and stir to combine well.
- Refrigerate for about 4-6 hours, stirring occasionally.

Per Serving: Calories: 325; Total Fat: 6.9g; Saturated Fat: 0.5g
Protein: 5.3g; Carbs: 69.4g; Fiber: 14.4g; Sugar: 52g

Pumpkin Quinoa Bowl

Serves: 6 / Preparation time: 15 minutes / Cooking time: 12 minutes

3½ cups filtered water

1¾ cups quinoa, soaked for 15 minutes and rinsed

14 ounces unsweetened coconut milk   1¾ cups homemade pumpkin puree

1 teaspoon ground cinnamon   ½ teaspoon ground ginger

Pinch of ground cloves   Pinch of ground nutmeg

3 tablespoons extra-virgin coconut oil   1 teaspoon stevia

1 teaspoon organic vanilla extract

- In a pan, add the water and quinoa over high heat and bring to a boil.
- Reduce the heat to low and simmer, covered for about 12 minutes or until all the liquid is absorbed.
- Stir in the remaining ingredients and remove from the heat.
- Serve warm.

Per Serving: Calories: 286; Total Fat: 11.3g; Saturated Fat: 8.3g
Protein: 7.8g; Carbs: 38.7g; Fiber: 6.1g; Sugar: 2.5g

Ginger Muffins

Serves: 6 / Preparation time: 15 minutes / Cooking time: 22 minutes

2 cups blanched almond flour

1 teaspoon baking soda

½ teaspoon ground ginger

1/8 teaspoon salt

½ cup organic honey

1 cup carrot, peeled and grated

½ cup unsweetened coconut shreds

½ teaspoon ground allspice

Pinch of ground cloves

3 organic eggs

½ cup coconut oil

2 tablespoons fresh ginger, grated

¾ cup raisins, soaked in water for 15 minutes and drained

- Preheat the oven to 350 degrees F. Grease 12 cups a large muffin tin.
- In a large bowl, add the flour, coconut shreds, baking soda, spices and salt and mix well.
- In another bowl, add the eggs, honey, and oil and beat until well combined.
- Add egg mixture into flour mixture and mix until well combined.
- Fold in the carrot, ginger and raisins.
- Place the mixture into the prepared muffin cups evenly.
- Bake for about 20-22 minutes or until a toothpick inserted in the center comes out clean.
- Remove from the oven and place the muffin tin onto a wire rack to cool for about 5 minutes.
- Carefully invert the muffins onto the wire rack to cool completely before serving.

Per Serving: Calories: 575; Total Fat: 41.4g; Saturated Fat: 19.7g
Protein: 11.8g; Carbs: 49.1g; Fiber: 5.9g; Sugar: 36g

Cranberry Bread

Serves: 8 / Preparation time: 20 minutes / Cooking time: 25 minutes

1 tablespoon honey

1 teaspoon active dry yeast

1/8 teaspoon salt

½ cup fresh orange juice

½ cup warm water

2 cups whole wheat flour

1/3 cup dried unsweetened cranberries

2-3 teaspoons fresh orange zest, grated

- In a bowl, dissolves the honey in the warm water.
- Sprinkle the yeast on top and set aside for about 5-10 minutes to proof.
- In the bowl of a stand mixer, add the flour, salt, cranberries and orange zest and mix well.
- Add the yeast mixture and orange juice and with the dough hook, mix until the dough comes together.
- Place the dough onto a lightly floured surface and with your hands, knead until a smooth dough ball is formed.
- Place the dough bowl into a greased glass bowl and turn to coat.
- With a plastic wrap, cover the bowl and set aside at a warm place for about 1-2 hours or until doubled in size.
- Place the dough onto a floured surface board and with your hands, knead until a dough ball is formed.
- With a lightly greased plastic wrap, cover the dough ball and set aside at a warm place for about 1-2 hours or until doubled in size.
- Preheat the oven to 450 degrees F. Place a 5-quart ceramic baking casserole with lid in the oven to preheat.
- Carefully, remove the casserole dish from the oven and line with a parchment paper.
- Place the dough into the casserole dish and cover with the lid.
- Bake for about 25 minutes or until a toothpick nested in the center comes out clean.
- Remove the bread pan from oven and place onto a wire rack to cool for about 5 minutes.
- Carefully invert the bread onto the wire rack and to cool completely before serving.
- Cut into desired sized slices and serve.

Per Serving: Calories: 135; Total Fat: 0.4g; Saturated Fat: 0.1g
Protein: 3.6g; Carbs: 29g; Fiber: 1.2g; Sugar: 4g

Apple Omelet

Serves: 1 / Preparation time: 10 minutes / Cooking time: 10 minutes

2 large organic eggs

2 teaspoons coconut oil, divided

¼ teaspoon ground cinnamon

1/8 teaspoon ground nutmeg

1/8 teaspoon organic vanilla extract

½ of large apple, cored and sliced thinly

1/8 teaspoon ground ginger

- In a bowl, add the eggs, vanilla extract and salt and beat until fluffy. Keep aside.
- In a nonstick frying pan, melt 1 teaspoon coconut oil over medium-low heat.
- Sprinkle the apple slices with spices evenly and place in the pan in a single layer.
- Cook for about 4-5 minutes, flipping once halfway through.
- Add the remaining oil in the skillet.
- Add the egg mixture over apple slices evenly.
- Tilt the pan to spread the egg mixture evenly and cook for about 3-4 minutes.
- Transfer the omelet into a plate and serve.

Per Serving: Calories: 284; Total Fat: 19.3g; Saturated Fat: 11g
Protein: 12.9g; Carbs: 17g; Fiber: 3.1g; Sugar: 12.5g

Spinach with Eggs

Serves: 4 / Preparation time: 15 minutes / Cooking time: 22 minutes

6 cups fresh baby spinach

4 organic eggs

2-3 tablespoons feta cheese, crumbled

2-3 tablespoons water

Salt and ground black pepper, as required

- Preheat the oven to 400 degrees F. Lightly, grease 2 small baking dishes.
- In a large frying pan, add spinach and water over medium heat and cook for about 3-4 minutes.
- Remove from heat and drain the excess water completely.
- Divide the spinach into prepared baking dishes evenly.
- Carefully, crack 2 eggs in each baking dish over spinach.
- Sprinkle with salt and black pepper and top with feta cheese evenly.
- Arrange the baking dishes onto a large cookie sheet.
- Bake for about 15-18 minutes.

Per Serving: Calories: 81; Total Fat: 5.1g; Saturated Fat: 1.7g
Protein: 7.6g; Carbs: 2g; Fiber: 1g; Sugar: 0.5g

S'

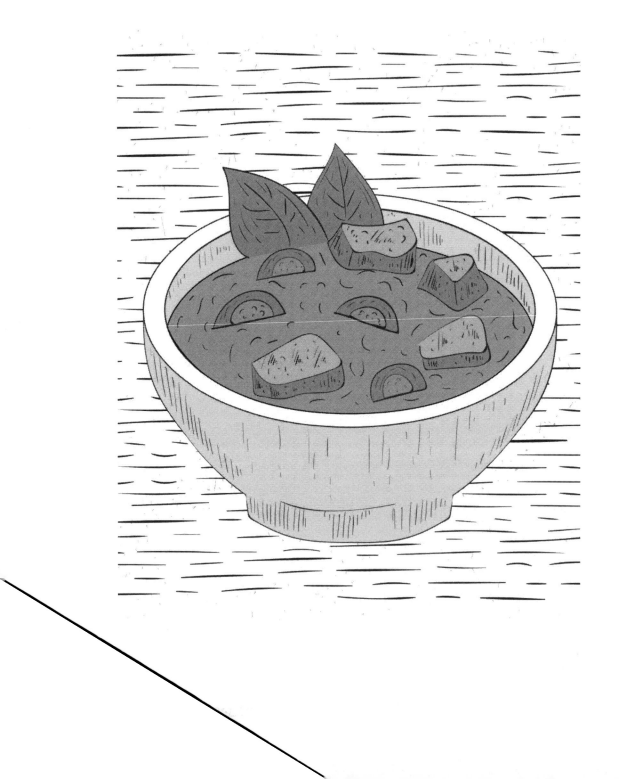

SOUPS & SALADS RECIPES

Contents

Broccoli Soup

Serves: 4 / Preparation time: 15 minutes / Cooking time: 35 minutes

1 tablespoon coconut oil

½ cup white onion, chopped

1 teaspoon ground turmeric

1 bay leaf

5 cups filtered water

1 small avocado, peeled, pitted and chopped

1 celery stalk, chopped

¼ teaspoon fresh ginger, grated

1 large head broccoli, cut into florets

Salt and ground black pepper, as required

1 tablespoon fresh lemon juice

- In a large soup pan, heat oil over medium heat and sauté the celery and onion for about 3-4 minutes.
- Add the ginger and turmeric and sauté for about 1 minute.
- Add remaining ingredients except avocado and lemon juice and bring to a boil
- Reduce the heat to medium-low and simmer, covered for about 25-30 minutes.
- Remove from the heat and set aside to cool slightly.
- In a blender, add the soup mixture and avocado in batches and pulse until smooth.
- Serve immediately with the drizzling of lemon juice.

Per Serving: Calories: 166; Total Fat: 13.5g; Saturated Fat: 5.1g
Protein: 3.2g; Carbs: 11g; Fiber: 5.7g; Sugar: 2.2g

Collard Greens Soup

Serves: 6 / Preparation time: 15 minutes / Cooking time: 50 minutes

2 tablespoons extra-virgin olive oil	1 large onion, chopped
Salt, as required	2 large leeks, sliced
2 tablespoons fresh ginger, minced	1 bunch collard greens, chopped
8 cups filtered water	1 tablespoon fresh lemon juice

- In a large soup pan, heat the oil over low heat and cook the onion and salt for about 20 minutes, stirring occasionally.
- Stir in the leeks and cook for about 10 minutes.
- Stir in the ginger and collard greens and cook for about 5 minutes.
- Add the water and bring to a boil over medium heat.
- Cook for about 10 minutes.
- Remove from the heat and set aside to cool slightly.
- In a blender, add the soup mixture and pulse until smooth.
- Return the soup in pan over medium heat and cook for about 5 minutes.
- Stir in the lemon juice and serve hot.

Per Serving: Calories: 112; Total Fat: 5.9g; Saturated Fat: 0.7g
Protein: 4.1g; Carbs: 15.1g; Fiber: 6.1g; Sugar: 2.3g

Cauliflower & Apple Soup

Serves: 5 / Preparation time: 20 minutes / Cooking time: 35 minutes

½ cup raw unsalted pistachios

2 cups carrots, peeled and sliced

1 teaspoon fresh ginger, minced

3 cups apples, cored and chopped roughly

Salt and ground black pepper, as required

2 tablespoons fresh cilantro, chopped

2 tablespoons extra-virgin olive oil

1 large onion, chopped

3 cups cauliflower, cut into small florets

1 teaspoon ground cumin

4 cups filtered water

- Preheat the oven to 400 degrees F.
- Place the pistachios onto a baking sheet and spread in an even layer.
- Bake for about 5-7 minutes or until toasted.
- Transfer the pistachios in a pan of water over medium heat and bring to a gentle boil.
- Simmer for about 35 minutes.
- Meanwhile, in a large soup pan, heat the oil over medium heat and sauté the carrot, onion and ginger for about 4-5 minutes.
- Add the cauliflower, apples and spices and cook for about 5 minutes, stirring occasionally.
- Add the water and bring to a boil.
- Reduce the heat to medium-low and simmer, covered for about 20 minutes.
- Remove from the heat and set aside to cool slightly.
- Drain the pistachios and set aside to cool slightly.
- Transfer the pistachios into a high-speed blender and pulse until creamy and smooth.
- Now, add the soup mixture in batches and pulse until smooth.
- Return the soup into the pan over medium heat and cook for about 2-3 minutes or until heated.
- Serve immediately with the garnishing of cilantro.

Per Serving: Calories: 198; Total Fat: 8.8g; Saturated Fat: 1.1g
Protein: 3.6g; Carbs: 30.8g; Fiber: 7.2g; Sugar: 19.2g

Lentil & Carrot Soup

Serves: 3 / Preparation time: 15 minutes / Cooking time: 30 minutes

6 small carrots, peeled and sliced

1 tablespoon mixed herbs

¼ cup split red lentils

1 teaspoon ground cumin

1/3 cup unsweetened coconut milk

3 tablespoons olive oil, divided

Salt and ground black pepper, as required

1 teaspoon mustard seeds

1 teaspoon ground turmeric

2 cups filtered water

- Preheat the oven to 355 degrees F.
- Arrange the carrot slices into a baking dish in a single layer.
- Drizzle with 1 tablespoon of oil and sprinkle with herbs, a pinch of salt and black pepper.
- Roast for about 25 minutes.
- Meanwhile, in a pan of the boiling water, add the lentils and cook for about 10 minutes.
- Drain the lentils well.
- In a large frying pan, heat the remaining oil over medium heat and sauté the mustard seeds, cumin and turmeric for about 30 seconds.
- In a blender, add the carrots, lentils, mustard seeds mixture, coconut milk and water and pulse until smooth.
- Transfer the soup mixture in a pan over medium heat and cook for about 4-5 minutes or until heated completely.
- Serve hot.

Per Serving: Calories: 290; Total Fat: 21.1g; Saturated Fat: 7.7g
Protein: 6.1g; Carbs: 8.5g; Fiber: 3g; Sugar: 6.3g

Salmon & Cabbage Soup

Serves: 4 / Preparation time: 15 minutes / Cooking time: 30 minutes

2 tablespoons extra-virgin olive oil

1 head cabbage, chopped

5 cups low-sodium bone broth

¼ cup fresh cilantro, minced

Ground black pepper, as required

1 onion, chopped

1 cup fresh mushrooms, sliced

2 (4-ounce) boneless salmon fillets, cubed

2 tablespoons fresh lemon juice

2 scallions, chopped

- In a large soup pan, heat the oil over medium heat and sauté the onion for about 5-6 minutes.
- Add the cabbage and mushrooms and sauté for about 5-6 minutes.
- Add broth and bring to a boil over high heat.
- Reduce the heat to medium-low and simmer for about 10 minutes.
- Add the salmon and cook for about 5-6 minutes.
- Stir in the cilantro, lemon juice and black pepper and cook for about 1-2 minutes.
- Serve hot with the topping of scallion.

Per Serving: Calories: 305; Total Fat: 10.8g; Saturated Fat: 1.6g
Protein: 39.4g; Carbs: 14.3g; Fiber: 5.5g; Sugar: 7.5g

Salmon & Quinoa Soup

Serves: 8 / Preparation time: 15 minutes / Cooking time: 1 hour 5 minutes

2 cups onions, chopped

2 tablespoons fresh ginger, chopped finely

1 cup quinoa, rinsed

16 ounces salmon fillets

1 cup fresh cilantro, chopped

2 scallions, chopped

1 cup celery, chopped

1 cup fresh shiitake mushrooms, sliced

8 cups low-sodium bone broth

6 cups fresh baby spinach

1 cup unsweetened coconut milk

- In a large soup pan, add the onions, celery, ginger, mushrooms, quinoa and broth and bring to a boil.
- Reduce the heat to low and simmer, covered for about 45 minutes.
- Arrange the salmon fillets over soup mixture.
- Simmer, covered for about 15 minutes.
- Stir in remaining ingredients except scallions and simmer for about 5 minutes.
- Serve hot with the garnishing of scallions.

Per Serving: Calories: 342; Total Fat: 12.2g; Saturated Fat: 7.1g
Protein: 36.3g; Carbs: 23g; Fiber: 4.2g; Sugar: 3.3g

Chicken Soup

Serves: 4 / Preparation time: 15 minutes / Cooking time: 25 minutes

1 tablespoon coconut oil

½ cup onion, chopped

1 tablespoon fresh thyme, chopped

½ teaspoon ground cumin

1¼ cups grass-fed cooked chicken, chopped

1¼ cups zucchini, chopped

2 tablespoons fresh lime juice

1 small carrot, peeled and chopped

1 celery stalk, chopped

1 tablespoon fresh rosemary, chopped

5 cups low-sodium bone broth

2 cups fresh spinach, torn

Ground black pepper, as required

1 teaspoon fresh lime zest, grated finely

- In a large soup pan, heat the oil over medium heat and sauté the carrot, onion and celery for about 8-9 minutes.
- Add the rosemary and spices and sauté for about 1 minute.
- Add the broth and bring to a boil over high heat.
- Reduce the heat to medium-low and simmer for about 5 minutes.
- Add the cooked chicken, spinach and zucchini and simmer for about 6-8 minutes.
- Stir in the black pepper and lime juice and remove from heat.
- Serve hot with the garnishing of lime zest.

Per Serving: Calories: 235; Total Fat: 5.2g; Saturated Fat: 3.4g
Protein: 39.5g; Carbs: 7.1g; Fiber: 2.6g; Sugar: 2.7g

Apple Salad

Serves: 4 / Preparation time: 15 minutes

For Salad

3 large apples, cored and sliced

6 cups fresh baby spinach

½ cup fresh cranberries

¼ cup unsalted walnuts, chopped

For Dressing

3 tablespoons extra-virgin olive oil

3 tablespoons fresh apple juice

2 tablespoons organic honey

2 tablespoons organic apple cider vinegar

- For salad: in a large bowl, add all the ingredients and mix.
- For dressing: in another bowl, add all the ingredients and beat until well combined.
- Place the dressing over salad and toss to coat well.
- Serve immediately.

Per Serving: Calories: 361; Total Fat: 15.8g; Saturated Fat: 1.9g
Protein: 3.8g; Carbs: 56.5g; Fiber: 6.5g; Sugar: 44g

Tropical Salad

1½ cups fresh pineapple, peeled and chopped

1½ cups mango, peeled, pitted and cubed   8 cups lettuce, torn

¼ cup fresh cranberries   ¼ cup fresh mint leaves, chopped

2 tablespoons fresh orange juice   Salt and ground black pepper, as required

- In a large serving bowl, add all the ingredients and toss to coat well.
- Cover and refrigerate to chill before serving.

Per Serving: Calories: 62; Total Fat: 0.4g; Saturated Fat: 0.1g
Protein: 1.1g; Carbs: 15.1g; Fiber: 2.2g; Sugar: 11g

Beans & Pomegranate Salad

Serves: 4 / Preparation time: 15 minutes / Cooking time: 10 minutes

2½ cups cooked white kidney beans

¼ cup scallion (green part), chopped finely

1 tablespoon fresh lime juice

¾ cup fresh pomegranate seeds

2 tablespoons fresh parsley, chopped

5 cups lettuce, torn

- In a large bowl, add all the ingredients except lettuce and toss to coat well.
- Divide lettuce onto serving plates and top with beans salad.
- Serve immediately.

Per Serving: Calories: 161; Total Fat: 0.2g; Saturated Fat: 0g
Protein: 10.7g; Carbs: 30.7g; Fiber: 13.3g; Sugar: 3.7g

Kale Salad

Serves: 6 / Preparation time: 15 minutes

For Dressing

2 tablespoons shallot, minced

¼ cup extra-virgin olive oil

¼ cup fresh lemon juice

Salt and ground black pepper, as required

For Salad

1½ pounds fresh Tuscan kale, trimmed and sliced thinly

14 ounces Brussels sprout, trimmed and grated finely

½ cup almonds, toasted and chopped

- For dressing: in another bowl, add all the ingredients and beat until well combined.
- For salad: in a large bowl, add all the ingredients and mix.
- Place the dressing over salad and toss to coat well.
- Serve immediately.

Per Serving: Calories: 207; Total Fat: 12.7g; Saturated Fat: 1.7g
Protein: 7.5g; Carbs: 20.3g; Fiber: 5.2g; Sugar: 2g

Mixed Veggies Salad

Serves: 12 / Preparation time: 20 minutes

For Salad

2 cups cauliflower, sliced thinly

2 cup carrots, peeled and sliced thinly

1 medium onion, sliced thinly in rings

2 cups cucumbers, sliced thinly

2 cups celery, sliced

10 cups fresh baby greens

For Vinaigrette

¾ cup extra-virgin olive oil

½ cup fresh parsley, minced

3 tablespoons balsamic vinegar

Salt and ground black pepper, as required

- For salad: in a large serving bowl, add all the ingredients and mix.
- For vinaigrette: in another bowl, add all the ingredients and beat until well combined.
- Place the vinaigrette over salad and gently toss to coat well.
- Serve immediately.

Per Serving: Calories: 131; Total Fat: 12.7g; Saturated Fat: 1.8g
Protein: 0.9g; Carbs: 4.9g; Fiber: 1.5g; Sugar: 2.3g

Tuna Salad

Serves: 4 / Preparation time: 20 minutes / Cooking time: 10 minutes

1 cup filtered water

½ cup low-fat plain yogurt

2 kiwifruit, peeled and chopped

1 cup mango, peeled, pitted and cubed

1 (6-ounce) can white tuna in water, drained and flaked

1 tablespoon unsweetened coconut, toasted

¾ cup uncooked instant brown rice

1-2 teaspoons fresh pineapple juice

1 cup pineapple, cubed

- In a pan, add the water over medium-high heat and bring to a boil.
- Add the rice and stir to combine.
- Reduce the heat to low and simmer, covered for about 10 minutes.
- Remove from the heat and set aside, uncovered for about 15 minutes.
- Refrigerate at least 1 hour or until cold.
- In a large bowl, add the rice, yogurt and pineapple juice and mix well.
- Cover the bowl and refrigerate for about 1-2 hours.
- In the bowl of rice mixture, add the fruit and gently, stir to combine.
- Garnish with coconut and serve immediately.

Per Serving: Calories: 277; Total Fat: 3.4g; Saturated Fat: 1.2g
Protein: 15.4g; Carbs: 46.7g; Fiber: 3.7g; Sugar: 15.3g

Salmon & Avocado Salad

Serves: 4 / Preparation time: 20 minutes / Cooking time: 15 minutes

2 (6-ounce) salmon fillets

Salt and ground black pepper, as required

2 avocados, peeled, pitted and cubed

¼ cup fresh cilantro, chopped

2 tablespoons extra-virgin olive oil

¼ cup coconut oil, melted

4 ounces fresh mushrooms, sliced

10 ounces lettuce, torn

2 tablespoons balsamic vinegar

- Preheat the broiler of oven. Line a baking sheet with a piece of foil.
- Coat the salmon fillets with 2 tablespoons of coconut oil and sprinkle with salt and black pepper lightly.
- Broil for about 15 minutes.
- Meanwhile, in a skillet, heat the remaining coconut oil over medium heat and sauté the mushrooms for about 4-5 minutes.
- Remove from the oven and with a sharp knife, cut the salmon into bite sized pieces.
- In a large bowl, add the salmon, mushrooms and remaining all ingredients and toss to coat well.
- Serve immediately.

Per Serving: Calories: 513; Total Fat: 45.7g; Saturated Fat: 17.7g
Protein: 19.6g; Carbs: 11.8g; Fiber: 7.5g; Sugar: 1.7g

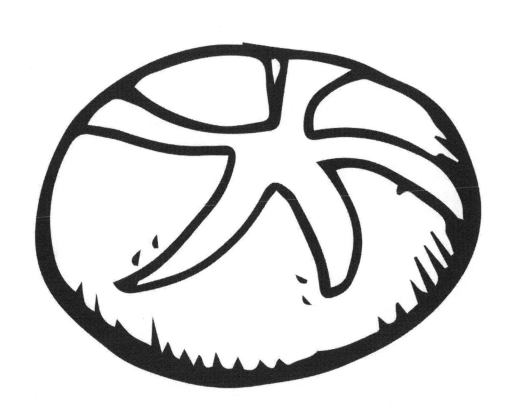

SNACKS & SIDES RECIPES

Contents

Almond Scones

Serves: 6 / Preparation time: 15 minutes / Cooking time: 20 minutes

1 cup almonds

¼ cup arrowroot flour

1 teaspoon ground turmeric

Ground black pepper, as required

¼ cup extra-virgin olive oil

1 teaspoon organic vanilla extract

1 1/3 cups almond flour

1 tablespoon coconut flour

1/8 teaspoon salt

1 organic egg

3 tablespoons raw honey

- Preheat the oven to 350 degrees F. Line a baking sheet with parchment paper.
- In a food processor, add the almonds and pulse until chopped roughly
- Transfer the chopped almonds into a large bowl with the flours and spices and mix well.
- In another bowl, add the remaining ingredients and beat till well combined.
- Add flour mixture into egg mixture and mix until well combined.
- Arrange a plastic wrap over cutting board.
- Place the dough over cutting board.
- With your hands, pat into about 1-inch thick circle.
- Carefully, cut the circle into 6 equal sized wedges.
- Arrange the scones onto the prepared baking sheet in a single layer.
- Bake for about 15-20 minutes.
- Remove from the oven and set aside to cool slightly.
- Serve warm.

Per Serving: Calories: 365; Total Fat: 29.2g; Saturated Fat: 3.3g
Protein: 10.2g; Carbs: 19.8g; Fiber: 5.7g; Sugar: 10.5g

Apple Leather

Serves: 4 / Preparation time: 15 minutes / Cooking time: 12 hours 25 minutes

1 cup filtered water

1 tablespoon ground cinnamon

8 cups apples, peeled, cored and chopped

2 tablespoons fresh lemon juice

- In a large pan, add the water and apples over medium-low heat and simmer for about 10-15 minutes, stirring occasionally.
- Remove from the heat and set aside to cool slightly.
- In a blender, add the apple mixture and pulse until smooth.
- Return the mixture into pan over medium-low heat.
- Stir in the cinnamon and lemon juice and simmer for about 10 minutes.
- Transfer the mixture onto dehydrator trays and with the back of spoon smooth the top.
- Set the dehydrator at 135 degrees F.
- Dehydrate for about 10-12 hours.
- Cut the apple leather into equal sized rectangles.
- Now, roll each rectangle to make fruit rolls.

Per Serving: Calories: 238; Total Fat: 0.9g; Saturated Fat: 0.1g
Protein: 1.3g; Carbs: 63.1g; Fiber: 11.7g; Sugar: 46.6g

Roasted Cashews

Serves: 16 / Preparation time: 10 minutes / Cooking time: 20 minutes

2 cups raw unsalted cashews

Pinch of salt

1 teaspoon extra-virgin olive oil

2 teaspoons organic honey

1 tablespoon fresh lemon juice

- Preheat the oven to 350 degrees F. Line a baking dish with the parchment paper.
- In a bowl, add all the ingredients and toss to coat well.
- Transfer the cashew mixture into the prepared baking dish and spread in a single layer.
- Roast for about 20 minutes, flipping once halfway through.
- Remove from the oven and set aside to cool completely before serving.
- You can preserve these roasted cashews in an airtight jar.

Per Serving: Calories: 104; Total Fat: 8.2g; Saturated Fat: 1.6g
Protein: 2.6g; Carbs: 6.4g; Fiber: 0.5g; Sugar: 1.6g

Banana Cookies

Serves: 7 / Preparation time: 15 minutes / Cooking time: 20 minutes

2 cups unsweetened coconut, shredded

3 medium bananas, peeled

½ teaspoon ground cinnamon

½ teaspoon ground turmeric

Pinch of salt and ground black pepper

- Preheat the oven to 350 degrees F. Line a cookie sheet with a lightly greased parchment paper.
- In a food processor, add all the ingredients and pulse until a dough like mixture forms.
- Make small balls from the mixture and place onto the prepared cookie sheet in a single layer.
- With your fingers, gently press down the balls to form the cookies.
- Bake for about 15-20 minutes or until golden brown.
- Remove from oven and place the cookie sheet onto a wire rack to cool for about 5 minutes.
- Carefully invert the cookies onto the wire rack to cool completely before serving.

Per Serving: Calories: 127; Total Fat: 7.8g; Saturated Fat: 68g
Protein: 1.4g; Carbs: 15.3g; Fiber: 3.5g; Sugar: 7.6g

Zucchini Chips

Serves: 2 / Preparation time: 15 minutes / Cooking time: 15 minutes

1 medium zucchini, cut into thin slices

1/8 teaspoon ground cumin

2 teaspoons extra-virgin olive oil

1/8 teaspoon ground turmeric

Pinch of salt

- Preheat the oven to 400 degrees F. Line 2 baking sheets with parchment papers.
- In a large bowl, add all the ingredients and toss to coat well.
- Transfer the mixture into prepared baking sheets and spread in a single layer.
- Bake for about 10-15 minutes.
- Serve immediately.

Per Serving: Calories: 57; Total Fat: 4.9g; Saturated Fat: 0.7g
Protein: 1.2g; Carbs: 3.4g; Fiber: 1.1g; Sugar: 1.7g

Citrus Cauliflower Rice

Serves: 4 / Preparation time: 15 minutes / Cooking time: 7 minutes

1 head cauliflower, cut into florets

2 tablespoons coconut oil, softened

1 teaspoon fresh lime zest, grated finely

1 tablespoon filtered water

½ cup fresh cilantro, chopped

2 tablespoons fresh lime juice

- In a food processor, add the cauliflower florets and pulse until it resembles like a rice consistency.
- In a microwave-safe dish, place the cauliflower rice and water.
- Cover the dish and microwave on High for about 7 minutes.
- Add the remaining ingredients and stir to combine well.
- Serve immediately.

Per Serving: Calories: 77; Total Fat: 6.9g; Saturated Fat: 5.9g
Protein: 1.4g; Carbs: 3.7g; Fiber: 1.8g; Sugar: 1.6g

Spiced Spinach

Serves: 4 / Preparation time: 15 minutes / Cooking time: 20 minutes

1 tablespoon extra-virgin olive oil

½ teaspoon fresh ginger, minced

½ teaspoon ground cumin

6 cups fresh spinach, chopped

1-2 tablespoons filtered water

1 red onion, chopped finely

1 teaspoon ground coriander

¼ teaspoon ground turmeric

Salt and ground black pepper, as required

- In a large skillet, melt the coconut oil over medium heat and sauté the onion for about 4-5 minutes.
- Add the ginger and spices and sauté for about 1 minute.
- Add the spinach, salt and black pepper and cook for about 2 minutes, stirring occasionally.
- Stir in the water and cook, covered for about 10 minutes.
- Uncover and stir fry for about 2 minutes.
- Serve warm.

Per Serving: Calories: 54; Total Fat: 3.8g; Saturated Fat: 0.5g
Protein: 1.7g; Carbs: 4.6g; Fiber: 1.7g; Sugar: 1.4g

Glazed Carrots

Serves: 4 / Preparation time: 15 minutes / Cooking time: 10 minutes

1 cup filtered water

1 pound carrot, peeled and cut into ½-inch slices

Pinch of salt

2 teaspoons fresh orange zest, grated

2 tablespoons fresh orange juice

1 tablespoon extra-virgin olive oil

2 tablespoons organic honey

Ground black pepper, as required

- In a pan, add the water, carrots and a pinch of salt and bring to a boil over high heat.
- Reduce the heat to medium and simmer for about 5 minutes.
- Drain the water well.
- In the same pan, add the remaining ingredients and carrot over medium heat and sauté for about 2-3 minutes or until glaze becomes slightly thick.
- Serve hot.

Per Serving: Calories: 113; Total Fat: 3.5g; Saturated Fat: 0.5g
Protein: 1g; Carbs: 20.9g; Fiber: 3g; Sugar: 14.9g

Creamy Broccoli

Serves: 2 / Preparation time: 15 minutes / Cooking time: 15 minutes

8 ounces broccoli, chopped

1 tablespoon coconut oil

1 onion, chopped

2 tomatoes, chopped

¼ teaspoon ground turmeric

¼ teaspoon ground cumin

½ teaspoon ground coriander

1 tablespoon unsweetened coconut, shredded

¼ cup filtered water

2 tablespoons unsweetened coconut milk

1 tablespoon fresh lemon juice

- In a pan of the boiling water, arrange a steamer basket.
- Place the broccoli in steamer basket and steam, covered for about 5 minutes.
- Drain the broccoli well.
- In a skillet, melt the oil over medium heat and sauté the onion for about 5 minutes.
- Add the remaining ingredients and bring to a gentle simmer.
- Stir in the broccoli and simmer for about 5 minutes.
- Serve hot.

Per Serving: Calories: 157; Total Fat: 8.7g; Saturated Fat: 7g
Protein: 5.1g; Carbs: 18.4g; Fiber: 6g; Sugar: 7.8g

Brussels Sprout

Serves: 4 / Preparation time: 15 minutes / Cooking time: 12 minutes

2 tablespoons extra-virgin olive oil

1 tablespoon cumin seeds

1 pound fresh Brussels sprouts, trimmed and halved

½ cup filtered water

1 tablespoon fresh ginger, minced

Salt and ground black pepper, as required

- In a skillet, heat the oil over medium heat and sauté the ginger and garlic for about 2 minutes.
- Add the cumin seeds, salt and black pepper and sauté for about 2 minutes.
- Stir in the Brussels sprouts and water and cook, covered for about 6-8 minutes.
- Serve hot.

Per Serving: Calories: 119; Total Fat: 7.8g; Saturated Fat: 1.2g
Protein: 4.3g; Carbs: 12g; Fiber: 4.6g; Sugar: 2.5g

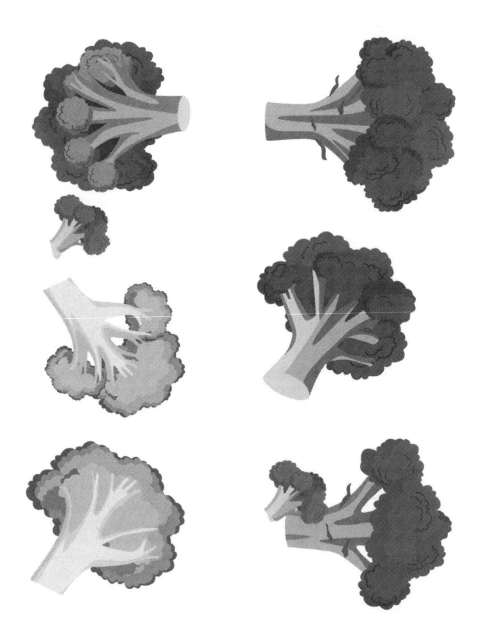

PLANT BASED MEAL RECIPES

Contents

Veggie Stew

Serves: 4 / Preparation time: 15 minutes / Cooking time: 21 minutes

2 tablespoons coconut oil

1 teaspoon ground turmeric

Salt and ground black pepper, as required

1 cup cabbage, shredded

2 large carrots, peeled and sliced

1 large onion, chopped

1 teaspoon ground cumin

1-2 cups filtered water, divided

1 bunch broccoli, chopped

2 teaspoons fresh ginger, grated

- In a large soup pan, melt coconut oil over medium heat and sauté the onion for about 5 minutes.
- Stir in the spices and sauté for about 1 minute.
- Add 1 cup water and bring to a boil.
- Simmer for about 10 minutes.
- Add the vegetables and enough water that covers the half of vegetable mixture and bring to a boil.
- Reduce the heat to medium-low and simmer, covered for about 10-15 minutes, stirring occasionally.
- Serve hot.

Per Serving: Calories: 129; Total Fat: 7.4g; Saturated Fat: 5.9g
Protein: 3.5g; Carbs: 15g; Fiber: 4.6g; Sugar: 5.4g

Beans & Carrot Stew

Serves: 5 / Preparation time: 15 minutes / Cooking time: 1 hour 20 minutes

2 tablespoons extra-virgin olive oil

1 teaspoon fresh ginger, chopped

1 cup dried adzuki beans, soaked for overnight, rinsed and drained

4 large carrots, peeled and sliced into ¾-inch pieces

2 tablespoons balsamic vinegar

¼ cup fresh parsley, minced

1 large yellow onion, chopped

3 cups filtered water

Salt and ground black pepper, as required

- In a large pan, heat the oil over medium heat and sauté the onion and ginger for about 2-3 minutes.
- Add the water and beans and bring to a boil.
- Reduce the heat to low and simmer, covered for about 45 minutes.
- Arrange the carrot slices over beans and simmer, covered for about 20-30 minutes.
- Stir in the vinegar, salt and black pepper and remove from heat.
- Serve hot with garnishing of parsley.

Per Serving: Calories: 217; Total Fat: 5.9g; Saturated Fat: 0.9g
Protein: 8.8g; Carbs: 33.8g; Fiber: 7.2g; Sugar: 4.2g

Chickpeas & Veggies Curry

Serves: 3 / Preparation time: 15 minutes / Cooking time: 25 minutes

¼ cup onion, chopped

1 (1-inch) piece fresh piece ginger, chopped

1 tablespoon coconut oil

½ teaspoon ground cumin

¼ teaspoon ground cinnamon

3 tablespoons almond butter

¾ cup zucchini, sliced

Salt and ground black pepper, as required

1 cup filtered water, divided

½ teaspoon ground coriander

½ teaspoon ground turmeric

½ cup unsweetened coconut milk

2 cups cooked chickpeas

¾ cup carrot, peeled and sliced

1 teaspoon fresh lime juice

¼ cup fresh cilantro, chopped

- In a blender, add onion, ginger, garlic and 2-3 tablespoons of water and pulse until smooth.
- In a pan, melt the coconut oil over medium heat and sauté the spices for about 30 seconds.
- Reduce the heat to medium-low.
- Add onion mixture and sauté for about 7-9 minutes.
- Add the coconut milk and almond butter and stir to combine well.
- Increase the heat to medium-high.
- Stir in broth, chickpeas, vegetables, red pepper flakes, salt and black pepper and bring to a boil for about 4 minutes.
- Reduce the heat to medium-low and simmer for about 5 minutes.
- Stir in the lime juice and cilantro and simmer for about 3-4 minutes.
- Serve hot.

Per Serving: Calories: 308; Total Fat: 16.4g; Saturated Fat: 5.6g
Protein: 11.5g; Carbs: 31.2g; Fiber: 7.9g; Sugar: 3.7g

Veggies Curry

Serves: 4 / Preparation time: 15 minutes / Cooking time: 25 minutes

2 teaspoons coconut oil

1 small white onion, chopped

1 tablespoon fresh ginger, chopped finely

3 carrots, peeled and cut into ¾-inch round slices

2 cups asparagus, trimmed and cut into 2-inch pieces

1 tablespoon curry powder

14 ounces unsweetened coconut milk

½ cup filtered water

2 cups fresh spinach, torn

1½ teaspoons balsamic vinegar

Salt and ground black pepper, as required

- In a large deep skillet, melt the coconut oil over medium heat and sauté the onion and ginger for about 5 minutes.
- Add the carrots, asparagus and curry powder and cook for about 3 minutes, stirring occasionally.
- Add the coconut milk and water and bring to a gentle simmer.
- Cook for about 5-10 minutes or until desired doneness of vegetables.
- Stir in the spinach and cook for about 3-4 minute.
- Stir in the vinegar, salt and black pepper and remove from heat.
- Serve hot.

Per Serving: Calories: 218; Total Fat: 16.3g; Saturated Fat: 14.4g
Protein: 3.9g; Carbs: 12.9g; Fiber: 3.8g; Sugar: 26.9g

Broccoli with Apple

Serves: 3 / Preparation time: 15 minutes / Cooking time: 16 minutes

1 tablespoon extra-virgin olive oil, divided

½ cup celery stalk, chopped

2 apples, cored and sliced

2 cups small broccoli florets

¼ cup filtered water

Salt and ground black pepper, as required

- In a large skillet, heat the oil over medium-high heat and stir fry the broccoli for about 4-5 minutes.
- Add the celery and stir fry for about 4-5 minutes.
- Stir in the water and cook for about 2-3 minutes.
- Stir in apple slices and cook for about 2-3 minutes.
- Stir in the salt and black pepper and remove from the heat.
- Serve hot.

Per Serving: Calories: 141; Total Fat: 5.2g; Saturated Fat: 0.7g
Protein: 2.2g; Carbs: 25.1g; Fiber: 5.5g; Sugar: 16.7g

Mushroom with Spinach

Serves: 2 / Preparation time: 15 minutes / Cooking time: 20 minutes

3 tablespoons coconut oil, divided

½ of red onion, sliced

Salt and ground black pepper, as required

3 cups fresh spinach, torn

1 cup fresh button mushrooms, sliced

½ teaspoon fresh lemon rind, grated finely

Pinch of ground nutmeg

½ tablespoon fresh lemon juice

- In a skillet, melt 1 tablespoon of the coconut oil over medium heat and cook the mushrooms for about 6-8 minutes.
- Transfer the mushrooms into a bowl and set aside.
- In the same skillet, melt the remaining oil over medium heat and sauté the onion and lemon rind for about 4-5 minutes.
- Stir in the spinach and cook for about 3-4 minutes.
- Stir in mushrooms and lemon juice and cook for about 1-2 minutes.
- Serve hot.

Per Serving: Calories: 207; Total Fat: 20.8g; Saturated Fat: 17.8g
Protein: 2.8g; Carbs: 5.6g; Fiber: 2g; Sugar: 2.1g

Stuffed Zucchini

Serves: 2 / Preparation time: 20 minutes / Cooking time: 45 minutes

2 medium zucchinis

½ cup onion, chopped

2 cups fresh Cremini mushrooms, cut into ½-inch pieces

1 cup plain whole wheat breadcrumbs

2 tablespoons fresh parsley, chopped

1 teaspoon dried basil

2 tablespoons extra-virgin olive oil

¼ cup low-fat feta cheese, crumbled

1 teaspoon dried oregano

Ground black pepper, as required

- Preheat the oven to 375 degrees F. Lightly, grease a baking sheet.
- Trim stem end from each zucchini and then, cut about 1/3 off the top of each horizontally.
- Carefully, cut a small horizontal sliver from the bottom of each zucchini.
- Chop the tops of zucchinis to ½-inch pieces.
- With a small paring knife, cut around inside of zucchini.
- With a small scooper, scoop out the flesh until the zucchini resembles a canoe.
- In a large skillet, heat the oil over medium heat and sauté the onion for about 2-3 minutes.
- Add the chopped zucchini tops and mushrooms and sauté for about 2 minutes.
- Remove from heat and stir in the breadcrumbs, feta cheese, parsley, oregano, basil and black pepper.
- Place the filling into each zucchini boat and press slightly.
- Arrange the zucchini boats onto the prepared baking sheet and bake for about 35-40 minutes.
- Serve warm.

Per Serving: Calories: 446; Total Fat: 23.5g; Saturated Fat: 7.1g
Protein: 22.7g; Carbs: 41g; Fiber: 7.7g; Sugar: 6.9g

Zucchini Noodles with Pesto

Serves: 3 / Preparation time: 15 minutes / Cooking time: 4 minutes

For Pesto

3 cups fresh basil leaves

Pinch of salt

¼ cup extra-virgin olive oil

¼ cup unsalted pine nuts, chopped roughly

Ground black pepper, as required

For Zucchini Noodles

1 tablespoon extra-virgin olive oil

2 large zucchinis, spiralized with blade C

- For pesto: in a food processor, add all the ingredients except oil and pulse until smooth.
- While motor is running, gradually, add oil and pulse until smooth.
- Transfer the pesto into a large bowl and set aside.
- In a large skillet, heat oil over medium heat and stir fry the zucchini noodles for about 3-4 minutes.
- Transfer the zucchini noodles in the bowl of pesto and gently, toss to coat well.

Per Serving: Calories: 303; Total Fat: 31.5g; Saturated Fat: 4g
Protein: 3.9g; Carbs: 6.5g; Fiber: 2.3g; Sugar: 2.7g

Lemony Veggie Noodles

Serves: 4 / Preparation time: 15 minutes / Cooking time: 12 minutes

1½ tablespoon extra-virgin olive oil   ¼ cup onion, chopped

1 large carrot, peeled and spiralized with Blade C

1 large yellow squash, spiralized with Blade C

1 large zucchini, spiralized with Blade C   2 tablespoon fresh lemon juice

Salt and ground black pepper, as required   ¼ cup scallion, chopped

- In a large skillet, heat the oil over medium heat and sauté the onion for about 4-5 minutes.
- Add the carrot and cook for about 2-3 minutes.
- Add the squash and zucchini and cook for about 3-4 minutes.
- Stir in the lemon juice, salt and black pepper and remove from the heat.
- Serve immediately with the garnishing of scallion.

Per Serving: Calories: 85; Total Fat: 5.6g; Saturated Fat: 0.9g
Protein: 2.4g; Carbs: 8.5g; Fiber: 2.6g; Sugar: 4.3g

Veggies in Cashew Sauce

Serves: 6 / Preparation time: 15 minutes / Cooking time: 20 minutes

For Sauce

4 cups filtered water

1 cup raw unsalted cashews

2 tablespoons fresh basil leaves, chopped

1 tablespoon fresh lemon juice

Salt and ground black pepper, as required

For Veggies

12 ounces fresh asparagus, trimmed and cut into 2-inch pieces

3 tablespoons extra-virgin olive oil

2 cups fresh Cremini mushrooms, chopped

3 medium zucchinis, sliced thinly

¼ cup pine nuts, chopped

- For cashew sauce: in a pan, add the water and bring to a boil.
- Remove from the heat and soak cashews in boiling water for about 30 minutes.
- Drain the cashews, reserving 1 cup of soaking water.
- In a blender, add the cashews, reserved water and remaining sauce ingredients and pulse until smooth.
- Set aside.
- In a large pan of the boiling water, add the asparagus and cook for about 2-3 minutes.
- Drain the asparagus well and set aside.
- In a large skillet, heat the oil over medium heat and sauté the mushrooms for about 5-6 minutes.
- Add the zucchini noodles and cashew sauce and cook for about 6-8 minutes.
- Add the asparagus and cook for about 2 minutes more.
- Serve hot with the garnishing of pine nuts.

Per Serving: Calories: 264; Total Fat: 21.8g; Saturated Fat: 3.5g
Protein: 7.4g; Carbs: 14.8g; Fiber: 3.3g; Sugar: 4.6g

Grilled Veggies

Serves: 6 / Preparation time: 20 minutes / Cooking time: 12 minutes

¼ cup olive oil

2 tablespoons organic honey

1 teaspoon ground cumin

3 small carrots, peeled and halved lengthwise

1 medium yellow squash, cut into ½-inch slices

1 medium zucchini, cut into ½-inch slices

1 medium red onion, cut into wedges

4 teaspoons balsamic vinegar

1 teaspoon dried oregano, crushed

Salt and ground black pepper, as required

1 pound fresh asparagus, trimmed

- In a small bowl, add all the ingredients except vegetables and mix well.
- In a large bowl, add 3 tablespoons marinade, reserving the remaining.
- Add vegetables and toss to coat well.
- Set aside, covered for about 1½ hours.
- Preheat the grill to medium heat. Grease the grill grate.
- Place the vegetables onto the grill grate in a single layer.
- Cover the grill and cook for about 8-12 minutes, flipping occasionally.

Per Serving: Calories: 139; Total Fat: 8.7g; Saturated Fat: 1.3g
Protein: 3g; Carbs: 15.4g; Fiber: 3.5g; Sugar: 10.3g

Veggie Kabobs

Serves: 4 / Preparation time: 20 minutes / Cooking time: 10 minutes

For Marinade

1 teaspoon fresh lemon peel, grated finely

1 teaspoon fresh basil, minced

2 tablespoons fresh lemon juice

1 teaspoon fresh rosemary, minced

2 tablespoons extra-virgin olive oil

Salt and ground black pepper, as required

For Veggies

1 large zucchini, cut into thick slices

8 large button mushrooms, quartered

1 head cauliflower, cut into florets

1 large red onion, cut into large cubes

- For marinade: in a large bowl, add all the ingredients and beat until well combined.
- Add the vegetables and toss to coat well.
- Cover the bowl and refrigerate to marinate for at least 8-10 hours.
- Preheat the grill to medium-high heat. Grease the grill grate.
- Remove the vegetables from bowl and discard any excess marinade.
- Thread the vegetables onto the pre-soaked wooden skewers.
- Place the skewers onto the grill and cook for about 8-10 minutes or until desired doneness, flipping occasionally
- Serve warm.

Per Serving: Calories: 115; Total Fat: 7.5g; Saturated Fat: 1.1g
Protein: 3.9g; Carbs: 11.4g; Fiber: 3.9g; Sugar: 5.4g

Quinoa & Veggie Wraps

Serves: 4 / Preparation time: 20 minutes / Cooking time: 10 minutes

For Filling

1 teaspoon extra-virgin olive oil

2 cups fresh shiitake mushrooms, chopped

1 teaspoon fresh lime juice

¼ cup scallion, chopped

1 cup cooked quinoa

1 teaspoon balsamic vinegar

Ground black pepper, to taste

For Wraps

8 medium butter lettuce leaves

¼ cup carrot, peeled and julienned

¼ cup cucumber, peeled and julienned

¼ cup unsalted walnuts, chopped

- For filling: in a skillet, heat the oil over medium heat and cook the mushrooms for about 5-8 minutes.
- Stir on the quinoa, lime juice and vinegar and cook for about 1 minute.
- Stir in the scallion and black pepper and immediately, remove from the heat.
- Set aside to cool.
- Arrange the lettuce leaves onto serving plates.
- Place quinoa filling over each leaf evenly and top with cucumber, carrot and walnuts.
- Serve immediately.

Per Serving: Calories: 260; Total Fat: 8.6g; Saturated Fat: 0.8g
Protein: 9.3g; Carbs: 39.8g; Fiber: 5.5g; Sugar: 3.4g

Lentil Burgers

Serves: 6 / Preparation time: 20 minutes / Cooking time: 17 minutes

1¾ cups plus 1 tablespoon filtered water, divided

¾ cup brown lentils, rinsed and drained

½ of large red onion, chopped finely

8 ounces fresh baby spinach

½ teaspoon ground cumin

½ cup unsalted walnuts, toasted and chopped finely

Olive oil cooking spray

2 teaspoons extra-virgin olive oil

1 tablespoon fresh lemon juice

Salt and ground black pepper, as required

1 cup whole-wheat plain breadcrumbs

- In a pan, add 1¾ cups of water and lentils over high heat and bring to a boil.
- Reduce the heat to medium-low and simmer, partially covered for about 30 minutes.
- Transfer the lentils into a bowl.
- Add the remaining water and with a potato masher, mash well.
- In a large nonstick skillet, heat the oil over medium heat and sauté the onion and lemon juice for about 6 minutes.
- Add the spinach, cumin and black pepper and cook for about 3 minutes.
- Transfer the spinach mixture into the bowl with mashed lentils.
- Add the breadcrumbs, walnuts and salt and mix until well combined.
- Refrigerate, covered for at least 1 hour or overnight.
- Preheat the grill to medium-high heat and lightly, grease the grill grate.
- Make 6 (4-inch) patties from the mixture.
- Coat the patties with the cooking spray from both sides.
- Grill the patties for about 3-4 minutes per side.
- Serve hot.

Per Serving: Calories: 224; Total Fat: 8.5g; Saturated Fat: 0.7g
Protein: 12g; Carbs: 27.5g; Fiber: 10.5g; Sugar: 1.7g

Quinoa with Green Beans

Serves: 4 / Preparation time: 15 minutes / Cooking time: 20 minutes

3 tablespoons extra-virgin olive oil, divided

1 cup dried quinoa, rinsed

1¾ cups filtered water

1 pound fresh green beans, trimmed and cut into 2-inch pieces

2 tablespoons fresh lemon juice

1 small onion, chopped

Salt and ground black pepper, as required

- In a pan, heat 1 tablespoon of oil over medium heat and sauté the onion for about 2-3 minutes.
- Add the quinoa and cook for about 1 minute, stirring continuously.
- Add salt, black pepper and water and bring to a boil.
- Reduce the heat to low and simmer, covered for about 15 minutes.
- Remove from the heat and set aside, covered for about 10 minutes.
- With a fork, fluff the quinoa.
- Meanwhile, in a pan of the boiling water, add the green beans and cook for about 4-5 minutes.
- Drain the green beans well.
- In a large serving bowl, mix together the quinoa and green beans.
- Drizzle with lemon juice and remaining oil and serve.

Per Serving: Calories: 291; Total Fat: 13.3g; Saturated Fat: 1.9g
Protein: 8.3g; Carbs: 37.2g; Fiber: 7.3g; Sugar: 2.5g

Quinoa & Spinach Pilaf

Serves: 3 / Preparation time: 15 minutes / Cooking time: 20 minutes

1 tablespoon extra-virgin olive oil, divided

1 teaspoon ground turmeric

¼ teaspoon ground cumin

1½ cups filtered water

½ cup scallions, sliced thinly

Salt and ground black pepper, as required

1 teaspoon fresh ginger, grated

¼ teaspoon ground coriander

1 cup golden quinoa, rinsed and drained

1½ cups fresh spinach leaves, chopped

¼ cup fresh lime juice

- In a medium pan, heat the oil over medium-high heat and sauté the ginger and spices for about 30 seconds.
- Add the quinoa and stir to combine.
- Add the water and bring to a boil.
- Reduce the heat to low and simmer, covered for about 15 minutes or until all the liquid is absorbed.
- Stir in the spinach and remove from heat.
- Set aside, covered for about 5 minutes.
- Stir in scallion, lime juice, salt and pepper and serve.

Per Serving: Calories: 263; Total Fat: 8.3g; Saturated Fat: 1.1g
Protein: 8.8g; Carbs: 39g; Fiber: 4.9g; Sugar: 0.5g

Rice & Cherries Pilaf

Serves: 8 / Preparation time: 20 minutes / Cooking time: 40 minutes

14 ounces low-sodium vegetable broth

1/3 cup filtered water

1 cup brown basmati rice

1 tablespoon curry powder

½ teaspoon ground turmeric

1/3 cup fresh lemon juice

3 tablespoons extra-virgin olive oil

3 tablespoons organic honey

1 tablespoon fresh ginger, minced

1 tablespoon fresh orange zest, grated

¾ cup celery stalk, chopped

½ cup scallion, chopped and divided

¾ cup dried unsweetened cherries, chopped roughly

1 cup fresh cherries, pitted and chopped

¾ cup unsalted almonds, chopped

- In a pan, add the broth, water, rice, curry powder and turmeric and mix well.
- Place the pan over medium-high heat and bring to a boil.
- Reduce the heat to low and simmer, covered for about 35 minutes.
- Remove from the heat and set aside, covered for about 5 minutes.
- With a fork, fluff the rice.
- In a large glass bowl, add the lemon juice, oil, honey, ginger and orange zest and mix well.
- Stir in the cooked rice, celery, ¼ cup of scallion and dried cherries.
- Serve immediately with the topping of fresh cherries, almonds and remaining scallion.

Per Serving: Calories: 265; Total Fat: 11g; Saturated Fat: 1.5g
Protein: 4.7g; Carbs: 38.9g; Fiber: 3.6g; Sugar: 14.2g

Rice Casserole

Serves: 3 / Preparation time: 15 minutes / Cooking time: 1 hour 5 minutes

1 teaspoon extra-virgin olive oil

1½ teaspoons ground turmeric

2 teaspoons raisins

1¼ cups low-sodium vegetable broth

1 tablespoon unsalted pine nuts, toasted and chopped

1 tablespoon fresh lemon juice

1 red onion, sliced thinly

9 ounces fresh brown mushrooms, sliced

½ cup brown rice, rinsed

¼ cup fresh cilantro, chopped

Ground black pepper, as required

- Preheat the oven to 400 degrees F.
- In an ovenproof pan, heat oil over medium heat and sauté the onion and turmeric for about 3-4 minutes.
- Add the mushrooms and stir fry for about 5-6 minutes.
- Stir in the raisins, rice and broth and immediately, transfer into oven.
- Bake for about 45-55 minutes or until desired doneness.
- Stir in the remaining ingredients and serve immediately.

Per Serving: Calories: 203; Total Fat: 4.7g; Saturated Fat: 0.6g
Protein: 6.4g; Carbs: 34.3g; Fiber: 2.9g; Sugar: 4.5g

Pasta Casserole

Serves: 6 / Preparation time: 15 minutes / Cooking time: 1 hour 10 minutes

For Sauce

1 cup sunflower seeds, shelled, soaked for 30 minutes, drained and rinsed

¼ cup low-sodium tamari   1½ cups filtered water

Pinch of ground black pepper

For Casserole

1 (14-ounce) package whole wheat fusilli pasta

2 tablespoons extra-virgin olive oil

3 cups fresh Brussels sprouts, trimmed and quartered

Ground black pepper, as required   1 cup filtered water

1 (14-ounce) package frozen spinach, thawed

- Preheat the oven to 400 degrees F. Grease large baking dish.
- For sauce: in a blender, add all the ingredients and pulse until smooth.
- Transfer the sauce into a bowl and set aside.
- In a pan of the boiling water, add the pasta and cook for about 8-10 minutes.
- Drain the pasta well and set aside.
- Meanwhile, in a large skillet, heat the oil over medium heat and cook the Brussels sprouts and black pepper for about 3-4 minutes.
- Add the water and cook for about 8-10 minutes.
- Stir in the spinach and cook for about 1 minute.
- Stir in the sunflower sauce and cook for about 1 minute.
- Stir in the cooked pasta and remove from the heat.
- Transfer the pasta mixture into prepared baking dish.
- Bake for about 35 minutes.
- Remove from the oven and set aside for about 5 minutes before serving.

Per Serving: Calories: 368; Total Fat: 10.8g; Saturated Fat: 1.1g
Protein: 13.7g; Carbs: 57.6g; Fiber: 9.7g; Sugar: 3.9g

Veggies Loaf

Serves: 8 / Preparation time: 15 minutes / Cooking time: 1 hour 10 minutes

1 tablespoon extra-virgin olive oil

1 teaspoon dried rosemary, crushed

2 large carrots, peeled and chopped

1¼ cups fresh button mushrooms, chopped

1¼ cups almond flour

2 large onions, chopped

1 cup unsalted walnuts, chopped

2 large celery stalks, chopped

5 large organic eggs

Salt and ground black pepper, as required

- Preheat the oven to 350 degrees F. Line 2 loaf pans with lightly greased parchment papers.
- In a large skillet, heat the oil over medium heat and sauté the onion for about 4-5 minutes.
- Add the rosemary and sauté for about 1 minute.
- Add the walnuts and vegetables and cook for about 3-4 minutes.
- Remove from heat and transfer the mixture into a large bowl.
- Set aside to cool slightly.
- In another bowl, add the eggs, flour, salt and black pepper and beat until well combined.
- Add the egg mixture into the bowl with vegetable mixture and mix until well combined.
- Divide the mixture into prepared loaf pans evenly.
- Bake for about 50-60 minutes or until top becomes golden brown.
- Remove from the oven and set aside for about 5-10 minutes before serving.

Per Serving: Calories: 282; Total Fat: 22.9g; Saturated Fat: 2.4g
Protein: 12.4g; Carbs: 11.4g; Fiber: 4.4g; Sugar: 3.8g

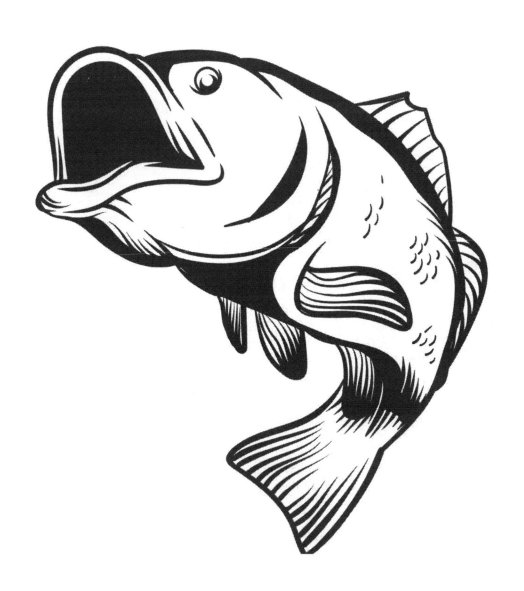

SEAFOOD RECIPES

Contents

Salmon with Salsa

Serves: 2 / Preparation time: 20 minutes / Cooking time: 8 minutes

For Salsa

¾ cup fresh pineapple, chopped

¾ cup mango, peeled, pitted and chopped

3 tablespoons red onion, chopped

2 tablespoons fresh cilantro, chopped

1 tablespoon fresh lemon juice

Ground black pepper, as required

For Salmon

2 (5-ounce) (1-inch thick) salmon fillets

Salt and ground black pepper, as required

1 tablespoon extra-virgin olive oil

- For salsa: in a bowl, add all the ingredients and toss to coat well.
- Refrigerate before serving.
- Season salmon with salt and black pepper.
- In a large skillet, heat the oil over medium-high heat.
- Place the salmon, skins side up and cook for about 4 minutes.
- Carefully change the side of fillets and cook for about 4 minutes more.
- Divide salsa onto serving plates alongside salmon fillets and serve.

Per Serving: Calories: 324; Total Fat: 16.2g; Saturated Fat: 2.4g
Protein: 28.6g; Carbs: 19g; Fiber: 2.2g; Sugar: 15g

Glazed Salmon

Serves: 4 / Preparation time: 15 minutes / Cooking time: 15 minutes

4 (6-ounce) salmon fillets

½ teaspoon fresh ginger, minced

1/3 cup fresh orange juice

1 scallion, chopped

¼ cup organic honey

¼ cup low-sodium tamari

- In a zip lock bag, add all ingredients and seal the bag.
- Shake the bag to coat the mixture with salmon.
- Refrigerate for about 30 minutes, flipping occasionally.
- Preheat the grill to medium heat. Grease the grill grate.
- Remove the salmon from the bag, reserving the marinade.
- Grill for about 10 minutes.
- Coat the fillets with reserved marinade and grill for 5 minutes more.

Per Serving: Calories: 309; Total Fat: 10.6g; Saturated Fat: 1.5g
Protein: 34.1g; Carbs: 21.4g; Fiber: 0.3g; Sugar: 19g

Teriyaki Salmon

Serves: 2 / Preparation time: 15 minutes / Cooking time: 11 minutes

¾ cup fresh pineapple juice

1 tablespoon balsamic vinegar

2 (4-ounce) salmon fillets

3 tablespoons low sodium tamari

1 tablespoon fresh ginger, chopped

- For teriyaki sauce: in a large bowl, add the pineapple juice, tamari, vinegar and ginger and mix until well combined.
- Heat a lightly greased nonstick skillet over medium-high heat and cook the salmon fillets for about 3 minutes per side.
- Add half of the teriyaki sauce and cook for about 5 minutes or until the desired doneness of salmon.
- Divide the salmon onto serving plates and serve with the topping of the remaining teriyaki sauce.

Per Serving: Calories: 230; Total Fat: 7.3g; Saturated Fat: 1.1g
Protein: 25.2g; Carbs: 15.4g; Fiber: 0.5g; Sugar: 9.5g

Salmon with Scallion

Serves: 4 / Preparation time: 15 minutes / Cooking time: 15 minutes

½ cup scallions, chopped

½ tablespoon extra-virgin olive oil

1/8 teaspoon red pepper flakes, crushed

Pinch of salt

4 (4-ounce) skin-on salmon fillets

- Preheat the oven to 450 degrees. Grease a roasting pan.
- In a small bowl, add the scallions, oil, red pepper flakes and a pinch of salt and mix well.
- In the bottom of the prepared roasting pan, arrange the salmon fillets, skin side down.
- Place the scallion mixture on top of each fillet evenly.
- Roast for about 15 minutes.
- Serve hot.

Per Serving: Calories: 169; Total Fat: 8.8g; Saturated Fat: 1.3g
Protein: 22.2g; Carbs: 1g; Fiber: 0.4g; Sugar: 0.3g

Honey Salmon

Serves: 2 / Preparation time: 15 minutes / Cooking time: 12 minutes

2 (6-ounce) salmon fillets

1/3 teaspoon ground turmeric, divided

2 large lemon slices

3 teaspoons organic honey, divided

Ground black pepper, as required

- In a zip lock bag, add salmon, ½ teaspoon of honey, ¼ teaspoon of turmeric and black pepper.
- Seal the bag and shake to coat well.
- Refrigerate to marinate for about 1 hour.
- Preheat the oven to 400 degrees F.
- Place the salmon fillets, skin-side up onto a baking sheet in a single layer and top with the marinade evenly.
- Bake for about 6 minutes.
- Carefully, change the side of fillets.
- Sprinkle with remaining turmeric and black pepper evenly.
- Place 1 lemon slice over each fillet and drizzle with the remaining honey.
- Bake for about 6 minutes.
- Serve hot.

Per Serving: Calories: 258; Total Fat: 10.5g; Saturated Fat: 1.5g
Protein: 33.1g; Carbs: 8.9g; Fiber: 0.1g; Sugar: 8.6g

Poached Salmon

Serves: 3 / Preparation time: 15 minutes / Cooking time: 12 minutes

1½ teaspoons fresh ginger, grated finely

1 tablespoon low-sodium tamari

1/3 cup fresh orange juice

3 (6-ounce) salmon fillets

- In a bowl, add all the ingredients except salmon and mix well.
- In the bottom of a large pan, place the salmon fillets.
- Place the ginger mixture over the salmon and set aside for about 15 minutes.
- Place the pan over high heat and bring to a boil.
- Reduce the heat to low and simmer, covered for about 10-12 minutes or until desired doneness.

Per Serving: Calories: 241; Total Fat: 10.6g; Saturated Fat: 1.5g
Protein: 33.5g; Carbs: 3.5g; Fiber: 0.1g; Sugar: 2.4g

Spicy Yogurt Salmon

Serves: 4 / Preparation time: 15 minutes / Cooking time: 14 minutes

¼ cup low-fat plain Greek yogurt

½ teaspoon ground cumin

Salt and ground black pepper, as required

½ teaspoon ground coriander

½ teaspoon ground turmeric

4 (6-ounce) skinless salmon fillets

- Preheat the broiler of oven. Grease a broiler pan.
- In a bowl, add all the ingredients except the salmon and mix well.
- Arrange salmon fillets onto prepared broiler pan in a single layer.
- Place the yogurt mixture over each fillet evenly.
- Broil for about 12-14 minutes.
- Serve hot.

Per Serving: Calories: 237; Total Fat: 10.8g; Saturated Fat: 1.7g
Protein: 33.9g; Carbs: 1.3g; Fiber: 0.1g; Sugar: 1g

Sweet & Tangy Salmon

Serves: 4 / Preparation time: 15 minutes / Cooking time: 12 minutes

1 tablespoon fresh ginger, grated finely

2 tablespoons organic honey

1 tablespoon low-sodium tamari

¼ cup scallion, chopped

4 tablespoons extra-virgin olive oil

2 tablespoons fresh lime juice

4 (4-ounce) boneless salmon fillets

- In a baking dish, add all the ingredients except the salmon and scallion and mix well.
- Add the salmon and coat with mixture generously.
- Refrigerate to marinate for about 40-45 minutes.
- Preheat the broiler of oven and arrange the rack in the top of the oven.
- Place the baking dish in the oven and broil for about 10-12 minutes.
- Divide the salmon fillets onto serving plates and top with the pan sauce.
- Serve with the garnishing of scallion.

Per Serving: Calories: 308; Total Fat: 21g; Saturated Fat: 3g
Protein: 22.4g; Carbs: 9.7g; Fiber: 0.2g; Sugar: 8g

Salmon Curry

Serves: 6 / Preparation time: 15 minutes / Cooking time: 35 minutes

6 (4-ounce) salmon steaks

3 tablespoons coconut oil, divided

3-4 green cardamom

1 onion, chopped finely

1 teaspoon red chili powder
¾ cup filtered water

¼ cup fresh cilantro, chopped

1½ teaspoons ground turmeric, divided

1 cinnamon stick

2 bay leaves

1½ teaspoons ginger paste

¾ cup low-fat plain Greek yogurt

- In a bowl, season the salmon with ½ teaspoon the turmeric and set aside.
- In a large skillet, melt 1 tablespoon of coconut oil over medium heat and cook the salmon for about 2-3 minutes per side.
- Transfer the salmon into a bowl.
- In the same skillet, melt the remaining oil over medium heat and sauté the cinnamon, green cardamom, whole cloves and bay leaves for about 1 minute.
- Add the onion and sauté for about 4-5 minutes.
- Add the garlic paste, ginger paste, green chilies and sauté for about 2 minutes.
- Reduce the heat to medium-low.
- Add remaining turmeric, red chili powder and salt and sauté for about 1 minute.
- Meanwhile, in a bowl, add the yogurt and water and beat until smooth.
- Now, reduce the heat to low and slowly, add the yogurt mixture, stirring continuously.
- Simmer, covered for about 15 minutes.
- Carefully, add the salmon fillets and simmer for about 5 minutes.
- Serve hot with the topping of cilantro.

Per Serving: Calories: 238; Total Fat: 14g; Saturated Fat: 6.9g
Protein: 25.3g; Carbs: 3.9g; Fiber: 0.7g; Sugar: 2g

Salmon Pasta

Serves: 8 / Preparation time: 15 minutes / Cooking time: 20 minutes

1 pound salmon fillet

16 ounces whole wheat penne pasta

2 teaspoons lemon zest, grated

2 tablespoons fresh lemon juice

Salt and ground black pepper, as required

½ cup fresh basil leaves, minced

2 tablespoons extra-virgin olive oil

- Preheat the oven to 350 degrees F. Grease a baking sheet.
- Season the salmon with salt and black pepper lightly.
- Arrange the salmon onto the prepared baking sheet and bake at for about 15-20 minutes.
- Meanwhile, in a pan of the boiling water, cook the pasta for about 8-10 minutes or until package's directions.
- Drain the pasta well and transfer into a large bowl.
- Add the basil, lemon zest, oil and lemon juice and toss to coat.
- Remove from oven and with a fork, flake the salmon into bite-sized pieces
- Add the salmon pieces into the bowl of pasta and gently, toss to coat.
- Serve immediately.

Per Serving: Calories: 296; Total Fat: 8g; Saturated Fat: 1g
Protein: 20g; Carbs: 40g; Fiber: 6g; Sugar: 0.1g

Herbed Sardines

Serves: 8 / Preparation time: 15 minutes / Cooking time: 6 minutes

1/3 cup olive oil

¼ cup fresh parsley, minced

Salt and ground black pepper, as required

16 fresh sardines, cleaned, rinsed and dried

¼ cup fresh thyme, minced

4-5 teaspoons lemon zest, grated

- In a bowl, add the oil, herbs, lemon zest, salt and black pepper and mix well.
- Stuff each sardine with herb mixture evenly.
- Preheat a gas grill to high heat. Grease the grill grate.
- Place the sardines onto the grill and cook for about 4–6 minutes, flipping once halfway through.
- Serve hot.

Per Serving: Calories: 313; Total Fat: 21.5g; Saturated Fat: 3g
Protein: 28.1g; Carbs: 1.3g; Fiber: 0.7g; Sugar: 0.1g

Sardines with Veggies

Serves: 4 / Preparation time: 20 minutes / Cooking time: 30 minutes

8 fresh sardines, cleaned, rinsed and dried

Salt and ground black pepper, as required

1 cup extra-virgin olive oil

2 carrots, peeled and cut into ¼-inch thick slices

1 small fennel bulb, trimmed and sliced thinly

1 celery stalk, cut into ¼-inch thick slices

1 yellow onion, sliced thinly

1 tablespoon fennel seed, crushed

3 bay leaves

- Preheat the oven to 300 degrees F.
- Season the sardines with salt and pepper lightly.
- Arrange the sardines in a 9x13-inch baking dish in a single layer.
- In a skillet, heat the oil over medium-high heat and cook the carrots, fennel bulb, celery, onion, fennel seeds, bay leaves and black pepper for about 10-12 minutes, stirring frequently.
- Remove from the heat and place the carrot mixture over the sardines evenly.
- Arrange a parchment paper over the surface of sardines and bake for about 25-30 minutes.
- Serve hot.

Per Serving: Calories: 646; Total Fat: 59.8g; Saturated Fat: 9.2g
Protein: 23.7g; Carbs: 10g; Fiber: 3.2g; Sugar: 2.7g

Lemony Sardines

Serves: 2 / Preparation time: 15 minutes / Cooking time: 10 minutes

1 onion, chopped finely

1 tablespoon fresh parsley, chopped

1 tablespoon extra-virgin olive oil

4 fresh sardines, cleaned, scaled and deboned

1 tablespoon fresh cilantro, chopped

1½ tablespoons fresh lemon juice

Salt and ground black pepper, as required

- In a bowl, add all the ingredients except sardines and mix well.
- Arrange the sardines in a shallow baking dish in a single layer and top each with the oil mixture evenly.
- Set aside for about 20 minutes, flipping once halfway through.
- Preheat a skillet over medium heat and cook the sardines for about 5 minutes per side.
- Serve hot.

Per Serving: Calories: 272; Total Fat: 20.5g; Saturated Fat: 4.4g
Protein: 18.1g; Carbs: 5.6g; Fiber: 1.3g; Sugar: 2.6g

Tuna with Relish

Serves: 6 / Preparation time: 20 minutes / Cooking time: 4 minutes

3 cucumbers, peeled and cut into a ¼-inch pieces

½ cup mixed olives, pitted and cut into a ¼-inch pieces

¼ cup fresh cilantro leaves, chopped

½ cup extra-virgin olive oil, divided   2 tablespoons fresh lemon juice

6 (8-ounce) (1-inch thick) tuna steaks

Salt and ground black pepper, as required

- For relish: in a bowl, add the cucumbers, olives, cilantro, ¼ cup of oil and lemon juice and mix.
- Season the tuna steaks with salt and black pepper lightly.
- In a large, heavy skillet. Heat 2 tablespoons of oil over high heat and sear 3 tuna steaks for about 1 minute.
- Flip and sear for about 40-50 seconds more.
- Transfer the tuna steaks onto a platter and cover with a piece of foil to keep warm.
- Repeat with the remaining oil and tuna steaks.
- Serve tuna steaks alongside the relish.

Per Serving: Calories: 409; Total Fat: 19g; Saturated Fat: 3g
Protein: 57.8g; Carbs: 6.3g; Fiber: 1.2g; Sugar: 2.6g

Sweet & Tangy Tuna

Serves: 4 / Preparation time: 15 minutes / Cooking time: 30 minutes

4 (4-ounce) tuna steaks

½ cup extra-virgin olive oil

2 tablespoons organic honey

Salt and ground black pepper, as required

¼ cup fresh lemon juice

1 teaspoon fresh ginger, minced

- Preheat the oven to 375 degrees F.
- Season the tuna steaks with salt and black pepper.
- In the bottom of a shallow baking dish, place about 2 tablespoons of oil.
- Arrange the tuna steaks over oil in a single layer.
- In a bowl, add the remaining oil, lemon juice, honey and ginger and mix well.
- Place the oil mixture over the tuna steaks evenly.
- Bake for about 30 minutes, basting with the oil mixture 2-3 times.
- Serve hot.

Per Serving: Calories: 371; Total Fat: 26.3g; Saturated Fat: 3.7g
Protein: 26.7g; Carbs: 8g; Fiber: 0.1g; Sugar: 9g

Citrus Glazed Tuna

Serves: 4 / Preparation time: 15 minutes / Cooking time: 12 minutes

¼ cup fresh orange juice

2 tablespoons olive oil

2 tablespoons fresh parsley, chopped

Ground black pepper, as required

2 tablespoons fresh lemon juice

2 tablespoons low-sodium tamari

½ teaspoon fresh oregano, chopped

4 (4-ounce) tuna steaks

- In a large non-reactive dish, add all the ingredients except the tuna steaks and mix well.
- Add the tuna steaks and coat with marinade generously.
- Cover the bowl and refrigerate for at least 30 minutes.
- Preheat grill for high heat. Lightly, grease the grill grate.
- Place the tuna steaks onto the grill and cook for about 5-6 minutes per side, flipping and basting with the marinade once halfway through.
- Serve hot.

Per Serving: Calories: 194; Total Fat: 8.1g; Saturated Fat: 1.1g
Protein: 27.3g; Carbs: 2.8g; Fiber: 0.3g; Sugar: 1.6g

Lemony Shrimp

Serves: 4 / Preparation time: 15 minutes / Cooking time: 7 minutes

1 small onion, chopped finely

1 tablespoon fresh ginger, minced

1 tablespoon fresh lemon zest, grated finely

1 teaspoon ground turmeric

½ cup extra-virgin olive oil

½ cup fresh lemon juice

1 pound shrimp, peeled and deveined

1 tablespoon coconut oil

- In a large bowl, add all the ingredients except shrimp and coconut oil and mix well
- Add the shrimp and coat with marinade generously.
- Cover and refrigerate to marinate for about 2-3 hours.
- Remove the shrimp from the bowl, reserving marinade.
- In a large nonstick skillet, melt the coconut oil over medium-high heat and stir fry the shrimp for about 3-4 minutes.
- Add the reserved marinade and bring to a boil, tossing occasionally.
- Cook for about 1-2 minutes.
- Serve hot.

Per Serving: Calories: 368; Total Fat: 30g; Saturated Fat: 6.8g
Protein: 23.7g; Carbs: 3.9g; Fiber: 0.9g; Sugar: 1.5g

Shrimp & Fruit Curry

Serves: 6 / Preparation time: 15 minutes / Cooking time: 15 minutes

2 teaspoons coconut oil, divided

1½ pounds shrimp, peeled and deveined

10 ounces pineapple, chopped

1 tablespoon red curry paste

½ cup onion, sliced thinly

1 mango, peeled, pitted and sliced

1½ cups unsweetened coconut milk

2 tablespoons fresh cilantro, chopped

- In a nonstick pan, melt 1 tablespoon of coconut oil over medium-high heat and sauté the onion for about 3-4 minutes.
- With a spoon, push the onion to the sides of the pan.
- Add the coconut oil and shrimp and cook for about 2 minutes per side.
- Add the remaining ingredients except cilantro and simmer for about 5-6 minutes.
- Serve hot with the garnishing of cilantro.

Per Serving: Calories: 322; Total Fat: 17.8g; Saturated Fat: 14.3g
Protein: 25.7g; Carbs: 19.3g; Fiber: 3.1g; Sugar: 14.3g

Shrimp with Yellow Squash

Serves: 2 / Preparation time: 15 minutes / Cooking time: 7 minutes

1 tablespoon extra-virgin olive oil

Ground black pepper, as required

2 medium yellow squashes, spiralized with Blade C

2 tablespoons fresh parsley, chopped

½ pound shrimp, peeled and deveined

1/3 cup low-sodium bone broth

- In a large skillet, heat the oil over medium heat and cook the shrimp and black pepper and for about 1 minute per side.
- Add broth and squash noodles and cook for about 4-5 minutes.
- Garnish with parsley and serve hot.

Per Serving: Calories: 207; Total Fat: 8.4g; Saturated Fat: 1.1g
Protein: 28.9g; Carbs: 6.8g; Fiber: 2.3g; Sugar: 3.4g

Shrimp Fajitas

Serves: 2 / Preparation time: 15 minutes / Cooking time: 17 minutes

2 tablespoons extra-virgin olive oil, divided

½ cup onion, sliced

1 teaspoon ground cumin

2 tablespoons fresh lime juice

4 ounces shrimp, peeled and deveined

1 cup fresh mushrooms, sliced

3 tablespoons fresh cilantro, chopped

2 whole-grain tortillas

- In a skillet, heat 1 tablespoon of oil over medium heat and cook the shrimp for about 2-3 minutes per side.
- Transfer the shrimp into a bowl and set aside.
- In the same skillet, heat the remaining oil over medium heat and sauté the onion for about 2-3 minutes.
- Add the mushrooms and cumin and cook for about 6-8 minutes.
- Stir in the shrimp, cilantro and lime juice and remove from the heat.
- Place the shrimp mixture over each tortilla and serve.

Per Serving: Calories: 345; Total Fat: 18.4g; Saturated Fat: 3.5g
Protein: 18.2g; Carbs: 29.5g; Fiber: 5.1g; Sugar: 3.9g

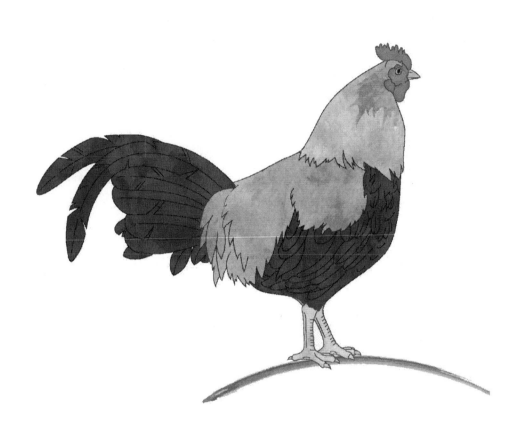

POULTRY RECIPES

Contents

Roasted Chicken

Serves: 6 / Preparation time: 15 minutes / Cooking time: 1 hour

½ teaspoon ground cumin   ½ teaspoon ground coriander

Salt and ground black pepper, as required

1 (3½-4-pound) grass-fed whole chicken, neck and giblets removed

4 large carrots, peeled and cut 1nto 2-inch pieces

2 unpeeled oranges, cut into wedges   ½ cup filtered water

- Preheat the oven to 450 degrees F.
- In a small bowl, mix together the spices.
- Rub the chicken with spice mixture evenly.
- Arrange the chicken in a large Dutch oven and place orange and carrot pieces around it.
- Add the water and cover the pan tightly.
- Roast for about 30 minutes.
- Uncover and roast for about 30 minutes.

Per Serving: Calories: 616; Total Fat: 37.9g; Saturated Fat: 10.8g
Protein: 55g; Carbs: 12g; Fiber: 2.7g; Sugar: 8g

Sweet & Sour Chicken Thighs

Serves: 6 / Preparation time: 15 minutes / Cooking time: 20 minutes

1 teaspoon fresh ginger, minced	½ cup fresh orange juice
1 tablespoon organic apple cider vinegar	2 tablespoons low-sodium tamari
¼ teaspoon ground cinnamon	Ground black pepper, as required
2 pounds grass-fed skinless, bone-in chicken thighs	

- For marinade: in a large bowl, add all the ingredients except chicken thighs and mix well.
- Add the chicken and coat with the marinade generously.
- Cover the bowl and refrigerate to marinate for about 2 hours.
- Remove the chicken thighs from the bowl, reserving marinade.
- Heat a large nonstick skillet, over medium-high heat and cook the chicken for about 5-6 minutes or until golden brown.
- Flip the side and cook for about 4 minutes.
- Add the reserved marinade and bring to a boil.
- Reduce the heat to medium-low and cook, covered for about 6-8 minutes or until sauce becomes thick.
- Serve hot.

Per Serving: Calories: 301; Total Fat: 11.2g; Saturated Fat: 3.1g
Protein: 44.2g; Carbs: 2.8g; Fiber: 0.2g; Sugar: 1.9g

Sweet & Spiced Chicken Breasts

Serves: 4 / Preparation time: 15 minutes / Cooking time: 20 minutes

1 teaspoon fresh ginger, minced

¼ cup extra-virgin olive oil

1 teaspoon ground cumin

4 (4-ounce) grass-fed skinless, boneless chicken breasts

1 cup fresh pineapple juice

1 teaspoon ground cinnamon

Salt, as required

- In a large Ziploc bag add all ingredients and seal it.
- Shake the bag to coat well.
- Refrigerate to marinate for about 1 hour.
- Preheat the grill to medium-high heat. Grease the grill grate.
- Place the chicken pieces onto the grill and cook for about 10 minutes per side.
- Serve hot.

Per Serving: Calories: 288; Total Fat: 16.9g; Saturated Fat: 3.4g
Protein: 25.7g; Carbs: 9g; Fiber: 0.6g; Sugar: 6g

Chicken with Veggies & Mango

Serves: 4 / Preparation time: 20 minutes / Cooking time: 20 minutes

2 tablespoons coconut oil

2 (8-ounce) grass-fed skinless, boneless chicken breasts, cut into slices

1 red onion, sliced thinly

1 ripe mango, peeled, pitted and cubed

1 large zucchini, sliced

2 tablespoons fresh lemon juice

¼ cup unsalted cashews, toasted

2 tablespoons fresh ginger, minced

1 cup small broccoli florets

1 cup fresh mushrooms, sliced

Salt and ground black pepper, as required

- In a large skillet, melt the coconut oil over medium-high heat and stir fry the chicken for about 4-5 minutes or until golden brown.
- With a slotted spoon, transfer chicken onto a plate.
- In the same skillet, add the onion and ginger and sauté for about 1-2 minutes.
- Add the mango, broccoli, zucchini and mushrooms and cook for about 5-7 minutes.
- Add the chicken, lemon juice, salt and black pepper and cook for about 4-6 minutes or until desired doneness.
- Serve with the topping of cashews.

Per Serving: Calories: 339; Total Fat: 15.5g; Saturated Fat: 8.4g
Protein: 29.9g; Carbs: 23.3g; Fiber: 3.9g; Sugar: 15.4g

Chicken with Rice

Serves: 6 / Preparation time: 20 minutes / Cooking time: 58 minutes

1 cup unsweetened coconut milk, divided
¼ teaspoon ground cumin
¼ teaspoon ground turmeric
1 pound grass-fed boneless, skinless chicken breasts, cut into 1-inch pieces
1½ cups brown basmati rice
1 large onion, sliced
6 ounces fresh green beans, trimmed and cut into ¼-inch pieces crosswise
¼ cup roasted unsalted cashews, chopped
2-3 tablespoons fresh lemon juice

1 teaspoon fresh ginger root, grated
¼ teaspoon ground coriander
Ground black pepper, as required

2 tablespoons extra-virgin olive oil
1 cinnamon stick

½ cup low-sodium bone broth
2 tablespoons fresh mint, chopped

- In a large bowl, add ½ cup of the coconut milk, ginger, ground spices and black pepper and mix well.
- Add the chicken and coat with the mixture generously.
- Cover the bowl and refrigerate for about 20-30 minutes.
- In a large pan of the boiling water, add the rice and cook for about 25 minutes.
- Drain the rice well.
- In a medium Dutch oven, heat the oil over medium-high heat and sauté the onion for about 5 minutes.
- Add the cinnamon stick and sauté for about 3 minutes.
- Reduce the heat to low.
- With a slotted spoon, transfer half of the onions onto a plate, leaving the cinnamon stick inside.
- Place the cooked rice over onion, followed by the green beans, half the cashews and chicken with marinade.
- Place the chicken broth and the remaining coconut milk on top and sprinkle with the reserved onions.
- Cover the pan tightly and cook for about 20 minutes or until the chicken and rice are cooked through.
- Stir in the lemon juice and remove from the heat.
- Serve with the topping of the remaining cashews and mint.

Per Serving: Calories: 509; Total Fat: 23.9g; Saturated Fat: 11.5g
Protein: 29.8g; Carbs: 45.1g; Fiber: 4.4g; Sugar: 3.2g

Chicken & Olives Stew

Serves: 12 / Preparation time: 20 minutes / Cooking time: 1 hour

4 pounds grass-fed skinless, boneless chicken thighs, trimmed

Ground black pepper, as required

3 large onions, sliced thinly

2 fresh bay leaves

2 teaspoon ground coriander

2 (3-inch) cinnamon sticks

½ cup fresh lemon juice, divided

2 cups small green olives, pitted

1 cup fresh cilantro, chopped

¼ cup extra-virgin olive oil

2 tablespoons fresh ginger, grated

1 tablespoon ground turmeric

2 teaspoons ground cumin

4 teaspoons lemon zest, grated finely

4 cups low-sodium bone broth

3 cups cooked chickpeas

- Season the chicken thighs with black pepper evenly.
- In a large pan, heat the oil over medium-high heat and cook the chicken thighs in 2 batches for about 3 minutes per side.
- With a slotted spoon, transfer the chicken thighs into a bowl and set aside.
- In the same pan, add the onion over medium heat and sauté for about 5-6 minutes.
- Add the ginger, bay leaves and spices and sauté for about 1 minute.
- Add lemon zest, 1/3 cup the lemon juice and broth and bring to a boil.
- Reduce the heat to medium-low and simmer, covered for about 30 minutes.
- Add the cooked chicken, olives and chickpeas and stir to combine.
- Increase the heat to medium-high and cook for about 6-8 minutes, stirring occasionally.
- Stir in the remaining lemon juice and black pepper and remove from heat.
- Serve hot with the garnishing of cilantro.

Per Serving: Calories: 352; Total Fat: 13g; Saturated Fat: 3.1g
Protein: 44g; Carbs: 14.1g; Fiber: 3.4g; Sugar: 2.1g

Chicken Chili

Serves: 5 / Preparation time: 15 minutes / Cooking time: 35 minutes

3 tablespoons extra-virgin olive oil

½ of red onion, chopped

1 zucchini, sliced

3 cups cooked cannellini beans

2 cups grass-fed cooked chicken, shredded

1 tablespoon fresh oregano, minced

1 teaspoon ground turmeric

1 teaspoon ground cumin

Ground black pepper, as required

2 cups filtered water

1 cup low-sodium bone broth

¼ cup fresh cilantro, chopped

- In a large pan, heat the oil over medium-low heat and sauté the onion for about 10 minutes.
- Add the zucchini and cook for about 5 minutes.
- Add the remaining ingredients except cilantro and bring to a boil.
- Reduce the heat to low and simmer for about 20 minutes.
- Serve hot with the topping of cilantro.

Per Serving: Calories: 322; Total Fat: 10.4g; Saturated Fat: 1.7g
Protein: 30.6g; Carbs: 27.5g; Fiber: 8.5g; Sugar: 3.6g

Ground Chicken with Peas

Serves: 4 / Preparation time: 15 minutes / Cooking time: 20 minutes

3 tablespoons extra-virgin olive oil

2 onions, grinded to a paste

2 tomatoes, chopped finely

1 tablespoon ground coriander

1 teaspoon red chili powder

1 pound grass-fed lean ground chicken

1½ cups filtered water

1 teaspoon garam masala powder

2 bay leaves

1 tablespoon ginger paste

1 tablespoon ground cumin

1 teaspoon ground turmeric

Salt, as required

2 cups frozen peas

2 tablespoons fresh cilantro, chopped

- In a deep skillet, heat the oil over medium heat and sauté the bay leaves for about 30 seconds.
- Add the onion paste and sauté for about 3-4 minutes.
- Add the ginger paste and spices and sauté for about 1-1½ minutes.
- Stir in the chicken and cook for about 4-5 minutes.
- Stir in peas and water and bring to a boil over high heat.
- Reduce the heat to low and simmer for about 5-8 minutes or until desired doneness.
- Stir in the cilantro and garam masala and remove from heat.
- Serve hot.

Per Serving: Calories: 350; Total Fat: 17.5g; Saturated Fat: 3.7g
Protein: 28.8g; Carbs: 21.3g; Fiber: 7g; Sugar: 7g

Ground Turkey with Spinach

Serves: 4 / Preparation time: 15 minutes / Cooking time: 17 minutes

1 tablespoon extra-virgin olive oil

½ of white onion, chopped

1 teaspoon fresh ginger, chopped finely

1 pound lean ground turkey

1 teaspoon ground coriander

1 teaspoon ground cumin

½ teaspoon ground turmeric

½ teaspoon ground cinnamon

Salt and ground black pepper, as required

1 pound fresh spinach leaves, chopped

1 teaspoon fresh lemon juice

- In a large skillet, heat the oil over medium heat and sauté onion for about 4 minutes.
- Add the ginger and sauté for about 1 minute.
- Add the turkey and spices and cook for about 6-8 minutes breaking into pieces with the spoon.
- Stir in the spinach and cook for about 4 minutes, stirring gently.
- Stir in the lemon juice and remove from heat.
- Serve hot.

Per Serving: Calories: 229; Total Fat: 12.2g; Saturated Fat: 3.1g
Protein: 25.8g; Carbs: 6.4g; Fiber: 3.1g; Sugar: 1.1g

Ground Turkey with Veggies

Serves: 4 / Preparation time: 15 minutes / Cooking time: 23 minutes

2 tablespoons coconut oil

1 pound lean ground turkey

½ of head cauliflower, chopped

2 celery stalks, sliced

½ teaspoon ground turmeric

1 red onion, sliced

1 small head broccoli, chopped

3 carrots, peeled and sliced

2 tablespoons fresh thyme, chopped

Salt and ground black pepper, as required

- In a large skillet, melt the coconut oil over medium heat and sauté the onion for about 5 minutes.
- Add the turkey and cook for about 6-8 minutes, breaking into pieces with the spoon.
- Add the remaining ingredients and cook for about 8-10 minutes, stirring occasionally.
- Serve hot.

Per Serving: Calories: 284; Total Fat: 15.3g; Saturated Fat: 8.5g
Protein: 25.4g; Carbs: 13.9g; Fiber: 4.7g; Sugar: 5.3g

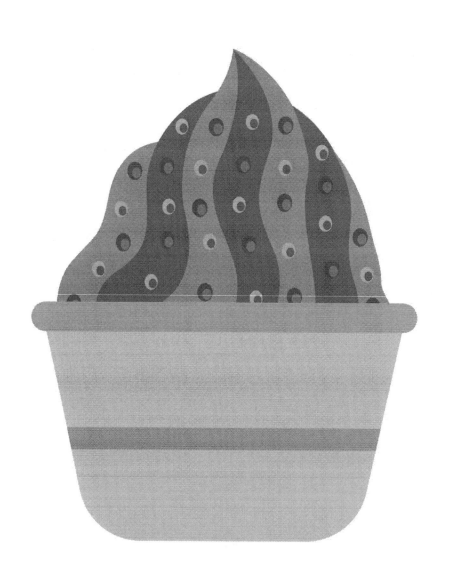

DESSERT RECIPES

Contents

Strawberry & Rhubarb Granita

Serves: 8 / Preparation time: 15 minutes / Cooking time: 10 minutes

1 cup fresh strawberries, hulled and halved

½ cup organic honey

1 tablespoon fresh mint leaves

3 cups rhubarb, sliced

2½ cups filtered water

- In a pan, add all the ingredients except mint over medium heat and cook for about 10 minutes, stirring occasionally.
- Through a strainer, strain the mixture by pressing gently.
- Discard the pulp of fruit.
- Transfer the strained mixture into a 13x9-inch glass baking dish.
- Freeze for about 20-30 minutes.
- Remove from freezer and with a fork scrap the mixture.
- Cover and freeze for about 1 hour, scraping after every 30 minutes.
- Serve with the garnishing of mint leaves.

Per Serving: Calories: 80; Total Fat: 0.2g; Saturated Fat: 0g
Protein: 0.6g; Carbs: 21g; Fiber: 1.3g; Sugar: 18g

Strawberry Sundae

Serves: 2 / Preparation time: 15 minutes

½ cup low-fat ricotta cheese

2 teaspoon fresh lemon juice

½ cup fresh strawberries, hulled and sliced

2 teaspoons organic vanilla extract

4 drops liquid stevia

2 teaspoon unsalted almonds, chopped

- In a bowl, add all the ingredients except strawberries and almonds and beat until smooth.
- In a serving glass, place ¼ of cheese mixture and top with ½ of strawberries.
- Top with ½ of remaining cheese mixture evenly.
- Repeat with another glass and remaining mixture.
- Garnish with almonds and serve immediately.

Per Serving: Calories: 122; Total Fat: 6g; Saturated Fat: 3.2g
Protein: 7.8g; Carbs: 7g; Fiber: 1g; Sugar: 2.7g

Mango Delight

Serves: 6 / Preparation time: 10 minutes

1½ cups fat-free plain Greek yogurt

4½ cups frozen mango, peeled, pitted and chopped

2 drops liquid stevia

- In a food processor, add all ingredients and pulse until smooth.
- Serve immediately.

Per Serving: Calories: 19; Total Fat: 0.6g; Saturated Fat: 0.1g
Protein: 7g; Carbs: 20g; Fiber: 2g; Sugar: 19g

Cranberry Mousse

Serves: 4 / Preparation time: 15 minutes / Cooking time: 2 minutes

1 cup unsweetened coconut milk

¼ cup organic honey

1 teaspoon organic vanilla extract

2 teaspoon fresh orange zest, grated finely

2 tablespoon fresh mint leaves, chopped finely

8 ounces fresh cranberries

3 tablespoons fresh orange juice

1 tablespoon unflavored gelatin

- In a high-speed blender, add the coconut milk and cranberries and pulse until smooth.
- Add the honey, orange juice and vanilla extract and pulse until well combined.
- Through a fine sieve, strain the mixture into a pan
- Place the pan over medium heat and cook for about 2 minutes.
- Remove from the heat.
- Slowly, add the gelatin, stirring continuously until dissolved completely.
- Fold in the orange zest and mint.
- Transfer the mixture into 4 serving bowls
- Refrigerate for about 1-4 hours or until set completely.

Per Serving: Calories: 212; Total Fat: 10g; Saturated Fat: 9g
Protein: 2.3g; Carbs: 27.4g; Fiber: 2.4g; Sugar: 21.6g

Pumpkin Pudding

Serves: 4 / Preparation time: 15 minutes

¾ cup homemade pumpkin puree

½ of avocado, peeled, pitted and chopped

¼ cup almond butter

¼ teaspoon ground ginger

Pinch of salt

1 ripe banana, peeled and sliced

¼ cup organic honey

1 teaspoon ground cinnamon

¼ teaspoon ground nutmeg

1 teaspoon organic vanilla extract

- In a food processor, add all the ingredients and pulse until smooth.
- Divide the pudding into 4 serving bowls.
- Refrigerate for at least 2 hours before serving.

Per Serving: Calories: 166; Total Fat: 5.8g; Saturated Fat: 1.2g
Protein: 1.6g; Carbs: 30.9g; Fiber: 4.3g; Sugar: 22g

Banana Custard

Serves: 8 / Preparation time: 10 minutes / Cooking time: 25 minutes

14 ounces unsweetened coconut milk

3 organic eggs

2 ripe bananas, peeled and mashed

½ teaspoon organic vanilla extract

- Preheat the oven to 350 degrees F. Lightly, grease 8 (6-inch) custard glasses. Arrange the glasses in a large baking dish.
- In a large bowl, add all ingredients and mix until well combined.
- Divide the banana mixture in prepared glasses evenly.
- Pour the water in the baking dish, about halfway full.
- Bake for about 20-25 minutes.
- Serve warm.

Per Serving: Calories: 165; Total Fat: 13.6g; Saturated Fat: 11g
Protein: 3.5g; Carbs: 9.7g; Fiber: 1.9g; Sugar: 5.4g

Banana Mug Cake

Serves: 1 / Preparation time: 15 minutes / Cooking time: 2½ minutes

1½ tablespoon coconut flour

Pinch of salt

1 tablespoon unsweetened coconut milk

1 teaspoon fresh lime zest, grated finely

2 tablespoon unsweetened coconut, shredded

½ tablespoon organic baking powder

1 organic egg

1 tablespoon fresh lime juice

1 banana, peeled and mashed

- Lightly, grease a microwave-safe mug.
- In a bowl, mix together flour, baking powder and salt.
- In another bowl, add the egg, coconut milk, lime juice, lime zest and banana and beat until well combined.
- Add the flour mixture into banana mixture and mix until well combined.
- Fold in the coconut.
- Transfer the mixture into the prepared mug and microwave on High for about 2-2½ minutes.
- Remove from microwave and keep aside to cool slightly before serving.

Per Serving: Calories: 360; Total Fat: 16.1g; Saturated Fat: 11.8g
Protein: 10.9g; Carbs: 46g; Fiber: 13g; Sugar: 17g

Mini Cherry Cakes

Serves: 6 / Preparation time: 15 minutes / Cooking time: 20 minutes

¾ cup fresh cherries, pitted and chopped

1/3 cup organic honey, divided

¼ teaspoon baking soda

¼ cup extra-virgin olive oil

1 teaspoon organic almond extract

¼ teaspoon vanilla bean powder, divided

1¼ cups almond flour

Pinch of salt

2 organic eggs

- Preheat the oven to 350 degrees F. Grease 6 cups a muffin tin.
- In a bowl, add the cherries, 1/8 teaspoon of the vanilla bean powder and 2 tablespoons of honey and mix well.
- In a second bowl, mix together the flour, baking soda and salt.
- In a third bowl, add oil, eggs, almond extract and remaining honey and vanilla bean powder and beat until well combined.
- Add the flour mixture into egg mixture and mix until well combined.
- Place the cherry mixture into prepared muffin cups evenly and top with flour mixture evenly.
- Bake for about 20 minutes or until a toothpick inserted in the center comes out clean.
- Remove the muffin tin from oven and place onto a wire rack to cool for about 10 minutes.
- Carefully invert the cakes onto a platter to cool completely before serving.

Per Serving: Calories: 297; Total Fat: 21.5g; Saturated Fat: 2.5g
Protein: 7.2g; Carbs: 23.5g; Fiber: 2.9g; Sugar: 18g

Apple Crisp

Serves: 8 / Preparation time: 15 minutes / Cooking time: 40 minutes

For Filling

2 cups Granny Smith apples, peeled, cored and sliced thinly

1 cup Fuji apple, peeled, cored and sliced thinly

1 cup fresh cranberries

Pinch of ground cinnamon

Pinch of ground nutmeg

1 tablespoon fresh lemon juice

For Topping

1 cup almond flour

¼ cup dates, pitted and chopped finely

Pinch of salt

1/3 cup extra-virgin olive oil

¼ cup pecans, chopped finely

½ teaspoon ground cinnamon

3 tablespoons organic honey

- Preheat the oven to 375 degrees F. Grease a 9x9-inch baking dish.
- For filling: in a large bowl, add all the ingredients and toss to coat well.
- For topping: in another bowl, add all the ingredients and toss to coat well.
- In the bottom of prepared baking dish, place the apple mixture and top the topping mixture evenly.
- Bake for about 40 minutes or until top becomes golden brown.
- Remove from the oven and set aside to cool slightly.
- Serve warm.

Per Serving: Calories: 273; Total Fat: 18.6g; Saturated Fat: 2g
Protein: 3.9g; Carbs: 27.2g; Fiber: 5g; Sugar: 19g

Yogurt Cheesecake

Serves: 8 / Preparation time: 15 minutes / Cooking time: 35 minutes

2½ cups low-fat Greek yogurt

3 organic egg whites

¼ cup arrowroot starch

Pinch of salt

6-8 drops liquid stevia

1/3 cup cacao powder

1 teaspoon organic vanilla extract

- Preheat the oven to 35 degrees F. Grease a 9-inch cake pan.
- In a large bowl, add all the ingredients and mix until well combined.
- Place the mixture into prepared pan evenly.
- Bake for about 30-35 minutes.
- Remove from oven and let it cool completely.
- Refrigerate to chill for about 3-4 hours or until set completely.
- Cut into 8 equal sized slices and serve.

Per Serving: Calories: 74; Total Fat: 0.9g; Saturated Fat: 0.4g
Protein: 9.5g; Carbs: 8.5g; Fiber: 1.1g; Sugar: 3g

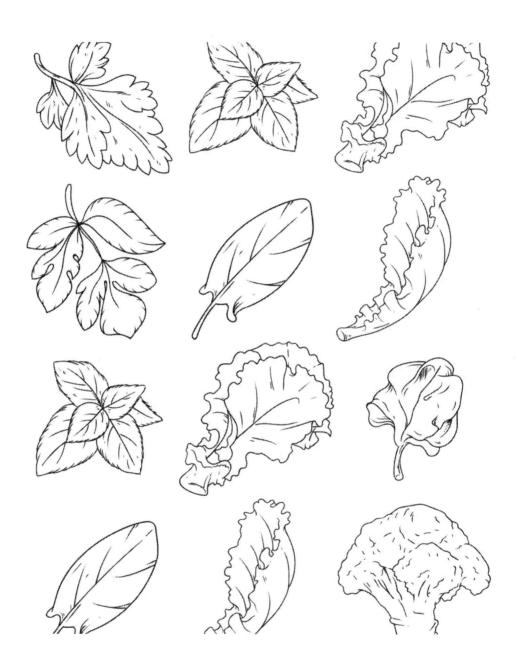

THE "DIRTY DOZEN" AND "CLEAN 15"

Every year, the Environmental Working Group releases a list of the produce with the most pesticide residue (Dirty Dozen) and a list of the ones with the least **chance of having residue (Clean 15). It's based on analysis from the U.S.** Department of Agriculture Pesticide Data Program report.

The Environmental Working Group found that 70% of the 48 types of produce tested had residues of at least one type of pesticide. In total there were 178 different pesticides and pesticide breakdown products. This residue can stay on veggies and fruit even after they are washed and peeled. All pesticides are toxic to humans and consuming them can cause damage to the nervous system, reproductive system, cancer, a weakened immune system, and more. Women who are pregnant can expose their unborn children to toxins through their diet, and continued exposure to pesticides can affect their development.

This info can help you choose the best fruits and veggies, as well as which ones you should always try to buy organic.

The Dirty Dozen

- Strawberries
- Spinach
- Nectarines
- Apples
- Peaches
- Celery
- Grapes
- Pears
- Cherries
- Tomatoes
- Sweet bell peppers
- Potatoes

The Clean 15

- Sweet corn
- Avocados
- Pineapples
- Cabbage
- Onions
- Frozen sweet peas
- Papayas
- Asparagus
- Mangoes
- Eggplant
- Honeydew
- Kiwi
- Cantaloupe
- Cauliflower
- Grapefruit

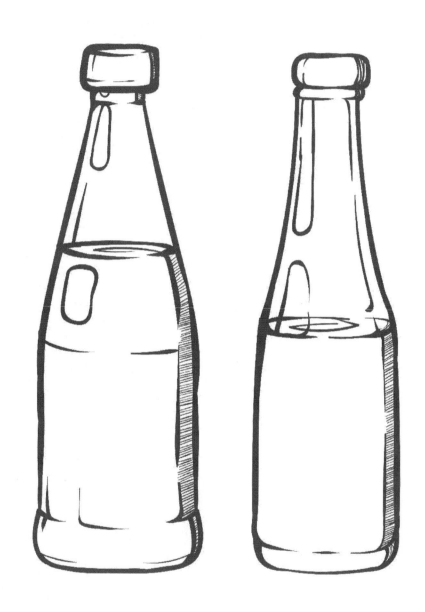

MEASUREMENT CONVERSION TABLES

Volume Equivalents (Dry)

US Standard	Metric (Approx.)
¼ teaspoon	1 ml
½ teaspoon	2 ml
1 teaspoon	5 ml
1 tablespoon	15 ml
¼ cup	59 ml
½ cup	118 ml
1 cup	235 ml

Weight Equivalents

US Standard	Metric (Approx.)
½ ounce	15 g
1 ounce	30 g
2 ounces	60 g
4 ounces	115 g
8 ounces	225 g
12 ounces	340 g
16 oz or 1 lb	455 g

Volume Equivalents (Liquid)

US Standard	US Standard (ounces)	Metric (Approx.)
2 tablespoons	1 fl oz	30 ml
¼ cup	2 fl oz	60 ml
½ cup	4 fl oz	120 ml
1 cup	8 fl oz	240 ml
1 ½ cups	12 fl oz	355 ml
2 cups or 1 pint	16 fl oz	475 ml
4 cups or 1 quart	32 fl oz	1 L
1 gallon	128 fl oz	4 L

Oven Temperatures

Fahrenheit (F)	Celsius (C) (Approx)
250°F	120°C
300°F	150°C
325°F	165°C
350°F	180°C
375°F	190°C
400°F	200°C
425°F	220°C
450°F	230°C

INDEX

Made in the USA
Monee, IL
22 June 2020